The Simulated Administrative Medical Office

Practicum Skills for Medical Assistants

powered by  SimChart®
for the medical office

The Simulated Administrative Medical Office

Practicum Skills for Medical Assistants

powered by SimChart®
for the medical office

Julie Pepper, CMA (AAMA)

Instructor
Medical Assistant Program
Chippewa Valley Technical College
Eau Claire, Wisconsin

ELSEVIER

ELSEVIER

1600 John F. Kennedy Blvd.
Ste 1800
Philadelphia, PA 19103-2899

THE SIMULATED ADMINISTRATIVE MEDICAL OFFICE

ISBN: 978-0-323-35393-9

Copyright © 2015 by Elsevier Inc.

Notices

Knowledge and best practice in this field are constantly changing. As new research and experience broaden our understanding, changes in research methods, professional practices, or medical treatment may become necessary.

Practitioners and researchers must always rely on their own experience and knowledge in evaluating and using any information, methods, compounds, or experiments described herein. In using such information or methods they should be mindful of their own safety and the safety of others, including parties for whom they have a professional responsibility.

With respect to any drug or pharmaceutical products identified, readers are advised to check the most current information provided (i) on procedures featured or (ii) by the manufacturer of each product to be administered, to verify the recommended dose or formula, the method and duration of administration, and contraindications. It is the responsibility of practitioners, relying on their own experience and knowledge of their patients, to make diagnoses, to determine dosages and the best treatment for each individual patient, and to take all appropriate safety precautions.

To the fullest extent of the law, neither the Publisher nor the authors, contributors, or editors, assume any liability for any injury and/or damage to persons or property as a matter of products liability, negligence or otherwise, or from any use or operation of any methods, products, instructions, or ideas contained in the material herein.

ISBN 978-0-323-35393-9

Senior Content Strategist: Jennifer Janson
Content Development Specialist: Heather Rippetoe
Product Specialist: Kate Gilliam
Content Development Manager: Ellen Wurm Cutter
Publishing Services Manager: Patricia Tannian
Senior Project Manager: Sharon Corell
Design Direction: XiaoPei Chen

Printed in the United States of America.

Last digit is the print number: 9   8   7   6   5   4   3

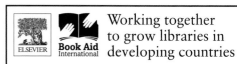

I would not be in the position to write this book if a dear friend had not told me about the medical assisting profession so many years ago. That conversation put me on this path. What a journey it has been, all thanks to Jill Lawrence!

There would be no reason for this book if SimChart for the Medical Office was never created. For that reason I also need to thank the team that started this wonderful project. It has been a joy to work with John Dolan, Kate Gilliam, Kevin Korinek, and Amy DeVore.

I could not have completed this work without the support of my family. Jeff, Megan, and Jon, you have been amazing throughout this whole process. I couldn't ask for more encouraging and patient people with whom to share all of this.

In memory of my mom, who was always so proud of my accomplishments.

Reviewers

Jeanne Lawo, RN, MSN
Clinical Manager
Saint Louis University
St. Louis, Missouri

Nikki Marhefka, M Ed, MT (ASCP), CMA (AAMA)
Program Director
Central Penn College
Summerdale, Pennsylvania

Tara Shepherd, CMA (AAMA)
Allied Health Director
Lead Instructor
Apollo Career Center
Lima, Ohio

Preface

In all healthcare professions there is a need to have an understanding of how electronic health records function. This book was written to address how the electronic health record functions in the administrative area of a medical clinic. It will take students on a 10-day journey of accomplishing tasks that are vital to the success of a medical clinic.

The purpose of *The Simulated Administrative Medical Office* is to simulate the tasks that an administrative medical assistant would perform while working in the front office of a medical practice. The student will complete tasks related to appointment scheduling, completion of common forms, inventory, correspondence, telephone messages, and coding and billing.

This textbook uses SimChart for the Medical Office as the basis for the practicum experience. The software allows students to become familiar with the functionality of an electronic health record. The skills learned while accomplishing those tasks will be transferable to whichever electronic health record (EHR) software students encounter in the real world. The tasks will help to build students' confidence in their abilities to use any EHR software.

SimChart for the Medical Office is web-based software that allows for instructor and student flexibility. Students can access the software wherever there is a computer and a connection to the Internet. Instructors can use the software for face-to-face classes, hybrid classes, or completely online classes.

Organization

The tasks of this text are organized over 10 days to simulate a 2-week practicum experience. Each day consists of four to five tasks that a medical assistant might be called on to perform during a day in an internship or practice. The tasks begin simply and then build on each other, gaining in complexity as familiarity with SimChart for the Medical Office is garnered.

Distinctive Features
- Images of important landing pages in SimChart for the Medical Office to get students started in the right place.
- Step-by-step instructions on each of the daily tasks to give students direction without completing the assignment for them.
- Professionalism boxes to provide students with the important soft skills training needed in the medical assisting profession.

Ancillaries

FOR THE STUDENT
- Direct access to SimChart for the Medical Office.
- Audio clips of patient messages to provide a realistic simulation of checking and responding to messages in a medical office.
- Other forms and documents to assist students with their daily front office duties.

FOR THE INSTRUCTOR

- Solutions to the daily tasks to provide guidance on what the student work should look like when completed in the EHR exercises.
- Commission on Accreditation of Allied Health Education Programs (CAAHEP) and Accrediting Bureau of Health Education Schools (ABHES) correlation grids to show how each task is tied to the standards of the field.

Contents

Day Seven

Day Eight

Day Nine

Day Ten

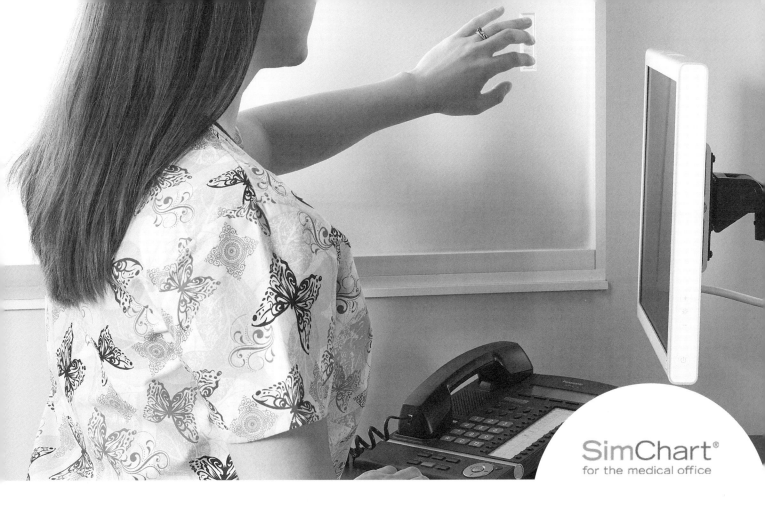

DAY ONE

Task 1.1
Preparing the Scheduling Matrix

Task 1.2
Rescheduling Appointments

Task 1.3
Scheduling an
Appointment for an Established Patient

Task 1.4
Scheduling New Patient Appointments

Task 1.5
Registering a New Patient

TASK 1.1

Preparing the Scheduling Matrix

For your first day at your internship at the Walden-Martin Family Medical Clinic, Jill, your mentor, wants you to get familiar with how the appointment schedule works. The appointment schedule is the basis for how the whole medical office functions *(Figure 1-1)*. Knowing how to use the electronic schedule will make you a valuable asset to any medical office.

The first step in creating a workable schedule is blocking out times that the providers are not available. There are times when all providers are not available to see patients, such as a monthly staff meeting, but there are also times that each individual provider would not be available. It is important that the matrix is set up correctly so that everyone knows which times are available for patients to be seen.

Your first task is to prepare the schedule for the next 6 months by blocking off times when the physicians will not be available for appointments. You will be blocking off times for the providers including lunch breaks, hospital and nursing home rounds, vacation times, and conferences.

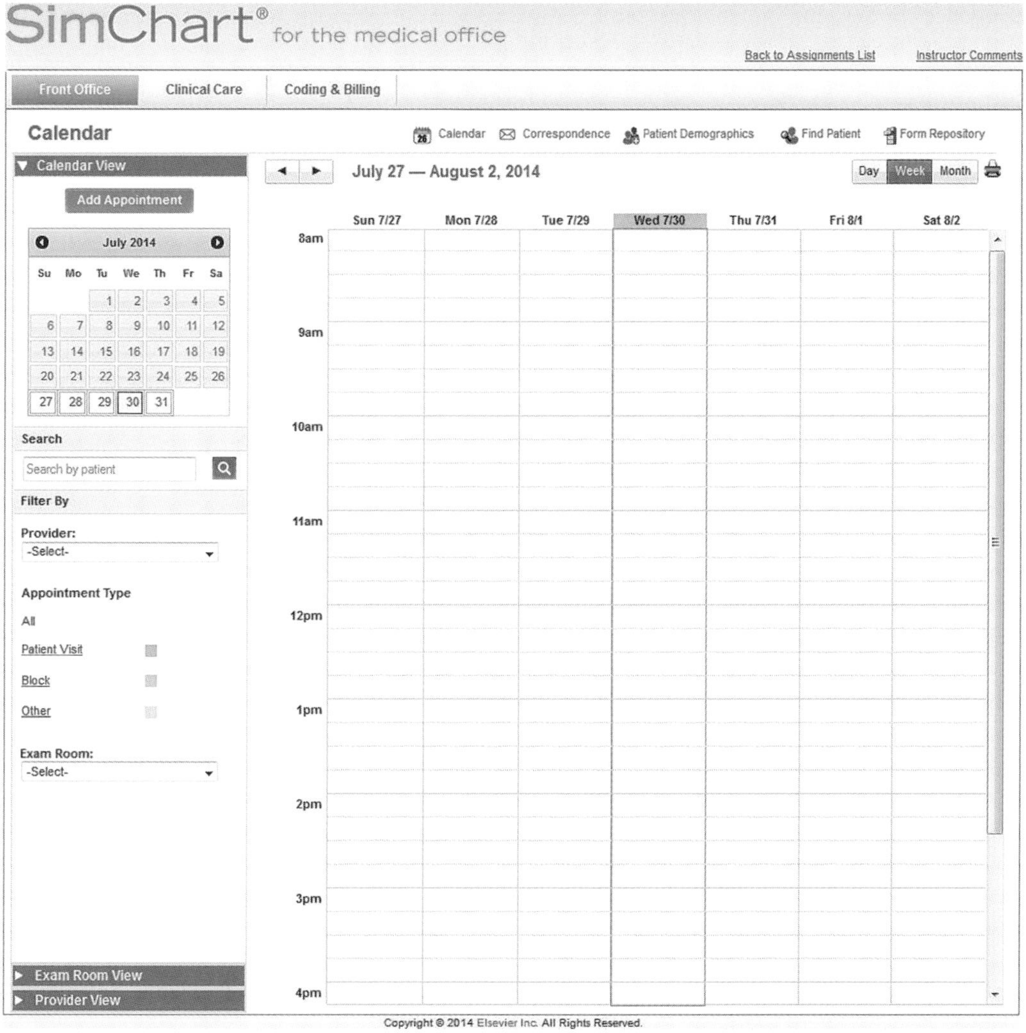

FIGURE 1-1   The appointment schedule.

✔ JAMES A. MARTIN, MD, SCHEDULE

LUNCH

Dr. Martin takes his lunch break daily from 12:30 to 1:30.

1. Click the **EHR Exercises** button to enter the simulation *(Figure 1-2)*.

2. Click the **Add Appointment** button. Note that all fields with an asterisk (*) are mandatory. You must have an entry in those fields in order to move forward.

3. In the **Appointment Type** field, select the **Block** radio button.

4. In the **Block Type** field, select **Lunch** from the drop-down menu.

5. In the **For** field, select **James A. Martin, MD** from the drop-down menu.

6. In the **Date** field, select today's date using the calendar picker.

7. Select a **Start Time** of **12:30 PM** and an **End Time** of **01:30 PM** from the drop-down menus.

8. This is an appointment that will be occurring every day, so the **Recurrence** box needs to be checked. In the **Recurrence Pattern** field, select the **Daily** radio button. In the **Recurrence Duration** field, use the calendar picker to select the **End By** radio button and choose the date that is 6 months from today's date.

9. Click the **Save** button. You may receive a message stating "New appointment conflicts with an existing appointment." Click the **OK** button. You will be rescheduling those appointments in a future task. You will see a confirmation message; click the **OK** button.

HOSPITAL ROUNDS

Dr. Martin does rounds at the hospital daily from 8:00 to 9:00 AM.

1. Click the **Add Appointment** button.

2. In the **Appointment Type** field, select the **Block** radio button.

FIGURE 1-2 EHR Exercises.

3. In the **Block Type** field, select **Other** from the drop-down menu and enter "Rounds" in the **Other** textbox.

4. In the **For** field, select **James A. Martin, MD** from the drop-down menu.

5. In the **Date** field, select today's date using the calendar picker.

6. Select a **Start Time** of **08:00 AM** and an **End Time** of **09:00 AM** from the drop-down menus.

7. This appointment will be occurring every day, so select the **Recurrence** box. In the **Recurrence Duration** field, select the **End By** radio button and choose the date that is 6 months from today's date using the calendar picker.

8. Click the **Save** button.

NURSING HOME ROUNDS

Dr. Martin makes rounds at the nursing home from 1:30 to 5:00 on Wednesdays.

1. Click the **Add Appointment** button.

2. In the **Appointment Type** field, select the **Block** radio button.

3. In the **Block Type** field, select **Other** from the drop-down menu and enter "Nursing Home Rounds" in the **Other** textbox.

4. In the **For** field, select **James A. Martin, MD** from the drop-down menu.

5. In the **Date** field, select the next Wednesday using the calendar picker.

6. Select a **Start Time** of **01:30 PM** and an **End Time** of **5:00 PM** from the drop-down menus.

7. This appointment will be occurring once a week, so select the **Recurrence** box. In the **Recurrence Duration** field, select the **End By** radio button and choose the date that is 6 months from today's date using the calendar picker.

8. Click the **Save** button.

VACATION

Dr. Martin will be taking vacation the first full week of next month. He will be gone Monday through Friday.

1. Click the **Add Appointment** button.

2. In the **Appointment Type** field, select the **Block** radio button.

3. In the **Block Type** field, select **Out-of-office** from the drop-down menu.

4. In the **For** field, select **James A. Martin, MD** from the drop-down menu.

5. In the **Date** field, select the Monday of the first full week of the next month using the calendar picker.

6. Select a **Start Time** of **08:00 AM** and an **End Time** of **06:00 PM** from the drop-down menus.

7. This appointment will be occurring daily, so select the **Recurrence** box.

8. In the **Recurrence Pattern** field, select the **Daily** radio button.

9. In the **Recurrence Duration** field, select the **End By** radio button and choose the Friday of the week of this vacation using the calendar picker.

10. Click the **Save** button.

CONFERENCE

Dr. Martin will be attending a full-day conference on innovations in diabetes treatments next Tuesday.

1. Click the **Add Appointment** button.

2. In the **Appointment Type** field, select the **Block** radio button.

3. In the **Block Type** field, select **Out-of-office** from the drop-down menu.

4. In the **For** field, select **James A. Martin, MD** from the drop-down menu.

5. In the **Date** field, select next Tuesday using the calendar picker.

6. Select a **Start Time** of **08:00 AM** and an **End Time** of **06:00 PM** from the drop-down menus.

7. Click the **Save** button.

You have now successfully set up the appointment matrix for Dr. Martin. Using what you have learned set up the appointment matrix for Dr. Julie Walden and Jean Burke, NP, using the information provided below.

 JULIE WALDEN, MD, SCHEDULE

1. Lunch break daily from 12:00 to 1:00 PM.

2. Hospital rounds daily from 8:30 to 9:30 AM.

3. Nursing home rounds weekly on Thursdays from 1:00 to 4:00 PM.

4. She will be taking vacation the second week of next month and will be gone Monday to Friday.

5. She will be presenting at the AAMA conference 2 weeks from today at 1:00 pm and will be gone for the afternoon.

 JEAN BURKE, NP, SCHEDULE

1. Lunch break daily from 11:30 to 12:30 PM.

2. Hospital rounds daily from 3:30 to 4:30 PM.

3. She will be taking vacation 3 weeks from Monday and will be gone Monday to Friday.

The appointment matrix is in place and now you can schedule appointments for patients. Jill lets you observe how she handles this, and now it is your turn to schedule appointments for an established patient. During your observation you notice that Jill was able to access the new appointment window by clicking within the appointment calendar. You can either use this method or click the Add Appointment button to complete the task below.

TASK 1.2

Rescheduling Appointments

Jill reminds you that when you were setting up the appointment matrix, you received a notification that the new appointment (lunch, rounds, vacation, etc.) conflicted with an existing appointment. You now need to reschedule those patient appointments that conflict with the newly established matrix.

 JAMES A. MARTIN, MD, SCHEDULE

1. To view Dr. Martin's schedule, select **James A. Martin, MD** from the **Provider** drop-down menu in the Calendar View section of the information panel on the left side of the screen *(Figure 1-3)*. Now the calendar will show only Dr. Martin's schedule.

2. Locate the patient appointments, shown in blue, that are scheduled at the same time as the blocked appointments, shown in pink.

3. Click on the patient appointment to view the details of that appointment. If this is a reoccurring appointment, you will be asked if you want to "Open this occurrence" or "Open the series."

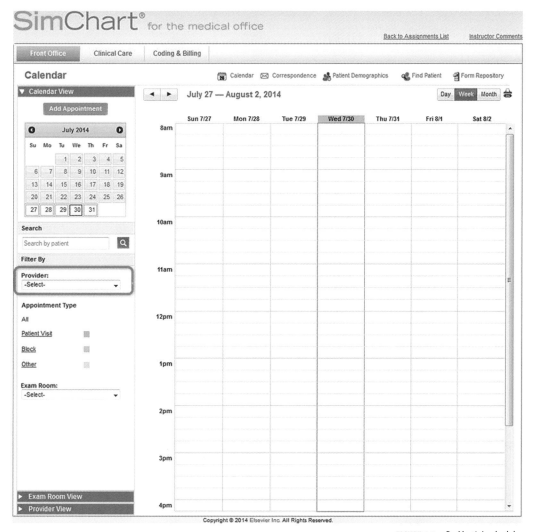

FIGURE 1-3 Dr. Martin's schedule.

4. Select the radio button next to **Open the Series** and then click the **OK** button. This will change all appointments scheduled at that time for this patient.

5. Adjust the start time and end time so that the appointment no longer conflicts with the blocked appointment (e.g., on the 5th of the month Quinton Brown has a 30-minute recurring appointment scheduled at 8:30 AM. This now conflicts with Dr. Martin's rounds. The new start time should be 9:00 AM, and the new end time should be 9:30 AM). Click the **Save** button.

6. You will see a confirmation message. Click the **OK** button. Continue to review the calendar and reschedule the appointments as necessary using the steps above.

✔ JULIE WALDEN, MD, SCHEDULE

1. To view Dr. Walden's schedule, select **Julie Walden, MD** from the Provider drop-down menu in the Calendar View section of the information panel on the left side of the screen. Now the calendar will show only Dr. Walden's schedule.

2. Locate the patient appointments, shown in blue, that are scheduled at the same time as the blocked appointments, shown in pink.

3. Review the calendar and reschedule the appointments as necessary.

✔ JEAN BURKE, NP, SCHEDULE

1. To view Jean Burke's schedule, select **Jean Burke, NP** from the Provider drop-down menu in the Calendar View section of the information panel on the left side of the screen. Now the calendar will show only Jean's schedule.

2. Locate the patient appointments, shown in blue, that are scheduled at the same time as the blocked appointments, shown in pink.

3. Review the calendar and reschedule the appointments as necessary.

TASK 1.3

Scheduling an Appointment for an Established Patient

Al Neviaser, DOB 06/21/1968, is an established patient of Dr. Martin. He has called in to schedule an appointment to have his blood pressure checked. This will be a follow-up visit that is 15 minutes in length. The patient has requested that this appointment be on a Friday during his lunch time, between 11:30 and 12:30 PM.

 ESTABLISHED PATIENT VISIT

1. Click the **Add Appointment** button or click within the appointment calendar.

2. In the **Appointment Type** field, select the **Patient Visit** radio button.

3. In the **Visit Type** field, select **Follow-up/Established Visit** from the drop-down menu.

4. In the **Chief Complaint** field, enter "Blood pressure check."

5. Select the **Search Existing Patients** radio button.

> ◎ **PROFESSIONALISM**
>
> It is always a good idea to search existing patient records even if the patient has stated that he or she is a new patient. This reduces the risk of creating duplicate records for patients.

6. Enter "Neviaser" in the **Last Name** field and click the **Go** button.

7. Verify the DOB, select the radio button next to his name, and click the **Select** button.

8. In the **Date** field, select Friday's date using the calendar picker.

9. Select a **Start Time** of **12:00 PM** and an **End Time** of **12:15 PM** from the drop-down menus.

10. Click the **Save** button. You will see a confirmation message.

11. Click the **OK** button. The appointment will appear on the calendar.

TASK 1.4

Scheduling New Patient Appointments

Now that you have experience in scheduling an appointment for an established patient, Jill would like you to schedule new patient appointments, which requires a bit more information. When scheduling an appointment for a new patient, some basic demographic information is obtained over the telephone; more complete information is obtained when the patient comes in for the appointment.

Angela Moore calls the clinic and would like to schedule an appointment with Dr. Walden. She states, "I have an itchy rash that's getting worse." According to the medical office's procedures, this type of complaint should be seen on the same day. A new patient visit is scheduled for 45 minutes *(Box 1-1)*.

✔ **NEW PATIENT VISIT**

1. Open Dr. Walden's schedule.

2. Find the first available 45-minute appointment for today and click on that time slot.

3. In the **Appointment Type** field, select the **Patient Visit** radio button.

4. In the **Visit Type** field, select **New Patient Visit** from the drop-down menu.

5. In the **Chief Complaint** field, enter "Itchy rash."

6. Select the **Search Existing Patients** radio button.

7. Enter "Moore" in the **Last Name** field and click the **Go** button.

8. If the patient's name does not exist in the system, click the **Cancel** button. A confirmation message will appear. Click the **OK** button.

9. Select the **Create New Patient** radio button.

10. Enter "Moore" in the **Last Name** field and "Angela" in the **First Name** field.

11. Using the calendar picker, enter 10/25/1992 in the **Date of Birth** field. The **Age** field will autopopulate.

12. Select the radio button next to **Female**.

BOX 1-1 Appropriate Appointment Times for Patients

NEW PATIENT VISIT
45 minutes
ANNUAL EXAM
45 minutes
FOLLOW-UP/ESTABLISHED VISIT
15 minutes
URGENT VISIT
15 minutes

```
AETNA                                1234 Insurance Way

MEMBER NAME: Moore, Angela

POLICY #: 654123789

GROUP #: WM753              EFFECTIVE DATE: 08/21/2013

CO-PAY: $25                              DRUG CO-PAY
SPECIALIST CO-PAY: $35                   GENERIC: $10
XRAY/LAB BENEFIT: $250               NAME BRAND: $50

         CLAIMS/INQUIRIES: 1-800-123-2222
```

FIGURE 1-4   Angela Moore's insurance card.

13. Enter "123-828-1886" in the **Home Phone** field.

14. Select **Julie Walden, MD** from the **Provider** drop-down menu.

15. Angela has given you her insurance information from her insurance card *(Figure 1-4)* and tells you that her SSN is 989-45-8888. Enter her insurance information and click the **Save** button. A confirmation message will appear. Click the **OK** button.

16. The **New Appointment** window will open and autopopulate with some of the information you just entered.

17. Use the calendar picker to choose today's date in the **Date** field.

18. Use the drop-down menu to choose the **Start Time**.

19. Use the drop-down menu to choose an **End Time** that is 45 minutes after the start time.

20. Click the **Save** button. You will see a confirmation message. Click the **OK** button. The appointment will appear on the calendar.

TASK 1.5

Registering a New Patient

When new patients arrive at the medical office, they are asked to provide more complete patient demographic information than what was obtained over the phone. They will complete a Patient Information Form to provide that information. Angela Moore has just arrived at the medical office and has completed her Patient Information Form *(Figure 1-5)*. You will need to enter the rest of her demographic information into the electronic health record.

 CHECKING IN ANGELA MOORE

1. Click the **Patient Demographics** icon.

2. Enter "Moore" in the **Last Name** field and click the **Search Existing Patients** button.

3. Angela's name should appear in blue. Click on **Angela**. There are three tabs for patient demographic information: **Patient**, **Guarantor**, and **Insurance**. All three have mandatory fields. Complete all of the mandatory fields (*) on the **Patient** tab and enter any other information that is supplied on the Patient Information Form.

4. Click on the **Guarantor** tab, complete all mandatory fields, and enter any other information that is supplied on the Patient Information Form.

5. Click on the **Insurance** tab, complete all mandatory fields, and enter any other information that is supplied on the Patient Information Form.

6. Click on the **Save Patient** button. You will see a confirmation message. Click the **Yes** button.

You have had a busy first day on your internship! You now have a firm handle on how the scheduling system works for setting up the appointment matrix, scheduling established and new patients, rescheduling patients, and registering new patients. Congratulations!

WALDEN-MARTIN
FAMILY MEDICAL CLINIC
1234 ANYSTREET ANYTOWN, ANYSTATE 1234
PHONE 123-123-1234   FAX 123-123-5678

PATIENT INFORMATION

PATIENT INFORMATION (Please use full legal name.)

Last name: _Moore_

First name: _Angela_

Middle initial: _M._

Medical record number: _____

Date of birth: _10/25/1992_

Age: _____

Sex: ☐ Male ☒ Female

SSN: _989-45-8888_

Emergency contact name: _Ruth Moore_

Mother's date of birth: _____

Mother's work phone: _____

Mother's SSN: _____

Language: _____

Address 1: _591 1st Avenue_

Address 2: _____

City: _Anytown_

State: _AL_

Zip: _12345-1222_

Email: _____

Home phone: _123-828-1886_

Driver's license: _____

Emergency contact phone: _123-858-1314_

Father's date of birth: _____

Father's work phone: _____

Father's SSN: _____

Race: _____

Ethnicity: _____

GUARANTOR INFORMATION (Please use full legal name.)

Relationship of guarantor to patient: ☒ Self ☐ Spouse ☐ Parent ☐ Other

Guarantor/account #: _____

Account number: _____

Last name: _____

First name: _____

Middle initial: _____

Date of birth: _____

Age: _____

Sex: _____

SSN: _____

Employer name: _Morgan's Office Supply_

School name: _____

Address 1: _____

Address 2: _____

City: _____

State: _____

Zip: _____

Email: _____

Home phone: _____

Cell phone: _____

Work phone: _123-552-9057_

FIGURE 1-5   Patient Information form for Angela Moore.

OTHER EMPLOYMENT INFORMATION

Father's employer: _____   Mother's employer: _____

Employer's address 1: _____   Employer's address 1: _____

Employer's address 2: _____   Employer's address 2: _____

City: _____   City: _____

State: _____   State: _____

Zip: _____   Zip: _____

PROVIDER INFORMATION

Primary provider: *Julie Walden MD*   Provider's address 1: *1234 Anystreet*

Referring provider: _____   Provider's address 2: _____

Date of last visit: *None*   City: *Anytown*

Phone: *123-123-1234*   State: *AL*

                                                Zip: *12345*

INSURANCE INFORMATION (If the patient is not the Insured party, please include date of birth for claims.)

PRIMARY INSURANCE

Insurance: *Aetna*   Claims address 1: *1234 Insurance Way*

Name of Policy Holder: *Angela Moore*   Claims address 2: _____

SSN: *989-45-8888*   City: *Anytown*

Policy/ID number: *654123789*   State: *AL*

Group Number: *WM 753*   Zip: *12345*

                                                Claims phone: *1-800-123-2222*

SECONDARY INSURANCE

Insurance: _____   Claims address 1: _____

Name of Policy Holder: _____   Claims address 2: _____

SSN: _____   City: _____

Policy/ID number: _____   State: _____

Group Number: _____   Zip: _____

                                                Claims phone: _____

"I hereby authorize direct payment of all insurance benefits otherwise payable to me for services rendered. I understand that I am financially responsible for all charges not covered by insurance for services rendered on my behalf to my dependents. I authorize the above providers to release any information required to secure payment of benefits. I authorize the use of this signature on all insurance submissions."

Signature: *Angela Moore*   Date: _____

FIGURE 1-5, cont'd

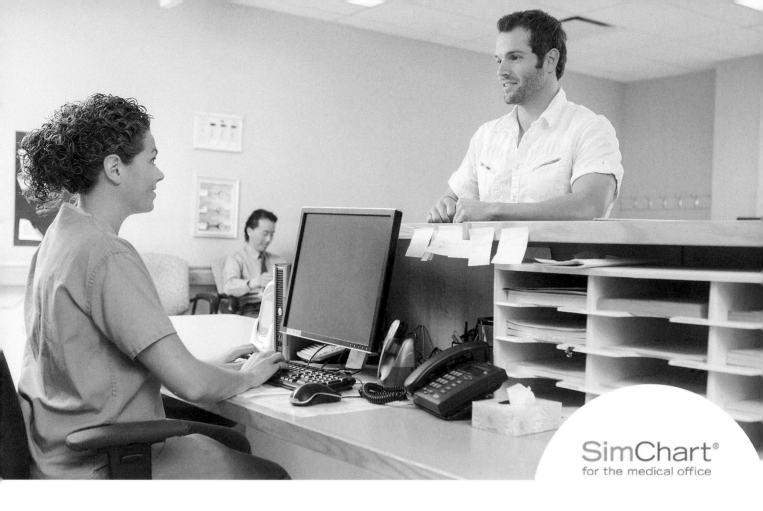

SimChart®
for the medical office

DAY TWO

TASK 2.1

Scheduling New Patient Appointments and Generating Appropriate Forms

Today you will continue to work with the schedule. Jill would like you to learn about how the electronic health record can be used to create forms and letters. Your first task is to schedule an appointment for a new patient and generate the forms needed for that patient.

The first call you take today is from Jon Wilson, who would like to schedule an annual examination with Dr. Martin. Jon is a new patient of the Walden-Martin Family Medical Clinic and has provided you with the following information:

Date of birth: 08/01/1986
Address:
987 Country Lane
Anytown, AL 12345-1234
Phone: 123-424-3098
Email: jwilson@wirefox.mail
Emergency contact: Elizabeth Wilson
Emergency contact phone: 123-424-3078
Langage: English
Race: White
Ethnicity: Not Hispanic or Latino
Employer: Anytown Technical College
Insurance:
MetLife
1234 Insurance Avenue
Anytown, AL 12345
Phone: 800-123-4444
Policyholder: Jon Wilson
Social Security number: 555-87-4298
Policy/ID number: SP12458679
Group number: 487956

Jon would like to have an appointment on a Wednesday, as this is his day off from work. Access Dr. Martin's schedule and find an available time for this appointment next Wednesday. Remember that a new patient visit as well as an annual examination will take 45 minutes.

Both New Patient Visit and Annual Exam are possible appointment types. In this situation, New Patient Visit would provide a better description.

✓ SCHEDULE A NEW PATIENT APPOINTMENT

1. Open Dr. Martin's schedule.

2. Find the first available 45-minute appointment for today and click on that time slot.

3. Enter the information necessary to schedule an appointment for this patient. The appointment will appear on the calendar (refer to Task 1.4).

Before moving on to the next step you will need to complete the demographic information for Jon Wilson. Using the information provided above, click the **Patient Demographics** icon *(Figure 2-1)*, perform a patient search, select the patient name displayed in blue, and complete the three tabs in the Patient Demographics window (refer to Task 1.5).

SimChart® for the medical office

Back to Assignments List   Instructor Comments

| Front Office | Clinical Care | Coding & Billing |

Calendar   Calendar   Correspondence   Patient Demographics   Find Patient   Form Repository

▼ Calendar View

Add Appointment

August 2014

Su	Mo	Tu	We	Th	Fr	Sa
					1	2
3	4	5	6	7	8	9
10	11	12	13	14	15	16
17	18	19	20	21	22	23
24	25	26	27	28	29	30
31						

Search

Search by patient

◄ ► August 3 — 9, 2014   Day Week Month

FIGURE 2-1 Patient Demographics icon.

✓ GENERATE APPROPRIATE FORMS

As Jon is a new patient of the clinic and has an appointment scheduled in the future, Jill informs you that several forms should be sent to Jon prior to his appointment. The Walden-Martin Family Medical Clinic sends all new patients a New Patient Welcome letter, the Notice of Privacy Practices, a Patient Bill of Rights, and a Medical Records Release form. Your next task is to prepare these documents to send to Jon Wilson.

NEW PATIENT WELCOME LETTER

1. Click on the **Correspondence** icon, click on **Letters**, and then click on **New Patient Welcome**.

2. Perform a **Patient Search** for Jon Wilson, verify the autopopulated information, and add any missing information.

3. Click the **Save to Patient Record** button.

You have successfully used the electronic health record to create a letter.

NOTICE OF PRIVACY PRACTICES

It is a Health Insurance Portability and Accountability Act (HIPAA) requirement that all patients receive the clinic's Notice of Privacy Practices. The Walden-Martin Family Medical Clinic chooses to send this to new patients prior to their appointment. You will prepare this notice to be included with the Welcome letter.

1. Click on the **Form Repository** icon, click on **Notice of Privacy Practice**.

2. Perform a **Patient Search** for Jon Wilson.

3. Click the **Save to Patient Record** button.

PATIENT BILL OF RIGHTS

The Walden-Martin Family Medical Clinic also sends new patients the Patient Bill of Rights document.

1. Locate the **Patient Bill of Rights** form and perform a **Patient Search**.

2. Click the **Save to Patient Record** button.

MEDICAL RECORDS RELEASE

It is also the policy at the Walden-Martin Family Medical Clinic to send new patients a Medical Records Release form so that any previous medical records can be sent to the clinic.

1. Locate the **Medical Records Release** form and perform a **Patient Search**.

2. Confirm the autopopulated information and complete the form for all of Jon's previous records.

3. Click the **Save to Patient Record** button.

To view the documents you have just created, click on the **Find Patient** icon and do a **Patient Search** for Jon Wilson. You will land on the Patient Dashboard of the electronic health record. By scrolling down the page, you will see the New Patient Welcome letter in the Correspondence section and the three forms you created in the Forms section. You can click on any of them to print them out if required by your instructor *(Figure 2-2)*.

FIGURE 2-2 New Patient Welcome letter documentation in the Correspondence section.

TASK 2.2

Creating Reminder Letters

Now that you are familiar with using letter templates, Jill would like you to create letters to remind patients of their upcoming appointments. You will be creating Appointment Reminder letters for the following patients:

- Quinton Brown
- Casey Hernandez
- Jana Green

1. Locate the **Appointment Reminder** letter template in **Correspondence**.

2. Perform a **Patient Search** for Quinton Brown.

3. Click on the next upcoming appointment from the **Select Appointments—Scheduled** list.

4. Click the **Save to Patient Record** button.

Repeat this task for Casey Hernandez and Jana Green.

TASK 2.3

Scheduling Urgent Appointments

Sometimes a patient needs to be seen on the same day, as soon as possible. Amma Patel, DOB 01/14/1988, has called in stating that she is 22 weeks pregnant and noticed some vaginal bleeding and cramping this morning. Dr. Walden is her physician. This type of situation usually warrants double booking the physician. Double booking happens when two patients are scheduled at the same time for the same physician.

1. Schedule Amma Patel for an Urgent Visit as soon as possible today with Dr. Walden even if it means double booking. Remember that the Chief Complaint is the reason that the patient is being seen (refer to Task 1.3).

◎ **PROFESSIONALISM**

When dealing with an upset patient on the telephone it is important for you to remain calm and collected. You should show the appropriate concern for the patient without upsetting the patient further. Empathy is important when dealing with a patient who is in a stressful situation.

TASK 2.4

Correcting Demographic Information

Scheduling appointments is one of the activities that is often done when you are responsible for answering the telephones in a medical office. Another is updating the patient's demographic information when there has been a change in address, employer, insurance, and so on. Jill feels that you are ready to take on this task. You will be using many of the skills you have already learned. You will need to locate established patients and then update the demographic information that has changed.

Update the following patient demographic information:

> Monique Jones
> Date of birth: 06/23/1985
> Employer: Anytown Attorneys
> Primary insurance:
> Aetna, 1234 Insurance Way
> Anytown, AL 12345
> Phone: 800-123-2222
> Policy/ID number: 4258796
> Group number: JK71133

1. Click on the **Patient Demographics** icon and search for Monique Jones, click on the patient name displayed in blue to update and edit the demographics.

2. After all three sections are complete and updated, click the **Save Patient** button.

Update the following patient demographic information:

> Diego Lupez
> Date of birth: 08/01/1982
> Address:
> 482 Grant Avenue
> Anytown, AL 12345
> Home phone: 123-838-0449

1. Using the information above, update the **Patient Demographics**.

2. After all three sections are complete and updated, click the **Save Patient** button.

TASK 2.5

Documenting Telephone Messages

Locate the **Telephone Messages** area on the companion Evolve website (Task 2.5). These are the nonurgent messages that came into the clinic during the hours in which the clinic was closed. Jill has asked you to listen to the messages and complete a Phone Message for each in the electronic health record.

1. Click on the **Correspondence** icon to locate **Phone Messages** in the information panel on the left side of the screen and perform a **Patient Search**.

2. Document the information accurately.

3. If a patient requests a specific time for an appointment, schedule the appointment as close as possible to the time requested by the patient. Indicate the date and time of the appointment in the **Action Documentation** section of the **Phone Message**.

4. Click the **Save to Patient Record** button.

You have learned some new aspects of the electronic health record today, and you will be able to apply those skills in the coming days. Well done!

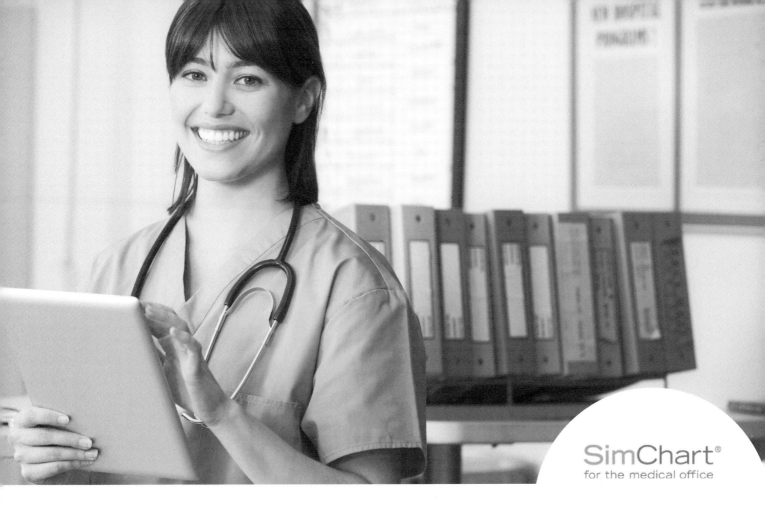

SimChart®
for the medical office

DAY THREE

Task 3.1
Risk Management

Task 3.2
Referral Form

Task 3.3
Written Communication

Task 3.4
Preparing a Superbill
and Posting to the Ledger

Task 3.5
Preparing an Insurance Claim

TASK 3.1

Risk Management

Today, Jill wants you to develop a better understanding of risk management in the medical office. You remember discussing risk management in school, but Jill would like you to see how those principles are applied in the actual clinic.

Risk is anything that may result in injury, illness, or financial loss to the clinic. Risk management involves policies and procedures that are in place to reduce those risks. You already followed some of the risk management policies when you prepared the appropriate forms for the new patient Jon Wilson by including the Notice of Privacy Practices and Medical Records Release forms with his New Patient Welcome letter. The Notice of Privacy Practices is required by HIPAA, and you are protecting the practice from a potential fine by documenting that the patient received it. By using the Medical Records Release form, you are protecting the office from an accusation of breach of confidentiality.

There are several other forms that are used in risk management, such as the Disclosure Authorization and the Incident Report.

✔ DISCLOSURE AUTHORIZATION

A Disclosure Authorization form should be signed if a patient wants someone else, such as a family member, to have access to the medical records or to allow health professionals to discuss the patient's condition with someone other than the patient.

Quinton Brown, DOB 02/24/1978, is an established patient of Dr. Martin. Quinton has had some recent health issues and would like his partner, Jon Angleston, to be able to have access to his records and discuss any issues with Dr. Martin. A Disclosure Authorization form will need to be completed.

> Jon Angleston
> Address:
> 4554 Browning Street
> Anytown, AL 12345

1. Find the **Disclosure Authorization** in the **Form Repository** and perform a **Patient Search**.

2. Review the autopopulated fields and complete all other required fields.

3. Click the **Save to Patient Record** button.

The Disclosure Authorization has now been saved to Quinton Brown's record and can be used to give information to Jon Angleston when he requests it.

After Amma Patel's pregnancy scare she decided that she would like her husband to be able speak to the doctor about her pregnancy. Complete the Disclosure Authorization form.

Gopal Patel
Address:
1346 Charity Lane
Anytown, AL 12345

1. Find the **Disclosure Authorization** in the **Form Repository** and perform a **Patient Search**.

2. Review the autopopulated fields and complete all other required fields.

3. Click the **Save to Patient Record** button.

✔ INCIDENT REPORT

An Incident Report is a document that is used to report any issues that affect patient or staff safety within the clinic. It provides documentation of what happened and can be used to develop safety measures so that the same problem does not occur again. The Incident Report form can be found in the Office Forms section of the Form Repository.

While you are sitting at the front desk, you witness a patient slip and fall as he enters the clinic. It is a rainy day, and the entryway floor is quite wet. Use the following information to complete the Incident Report:

Today's date and time:
Department: Family practice
Medical team: Dr. Martin
Patient reason for visit: Appointment
Immediate actions: Dr. Martin assessed patient injuries. Minor bruising
    found. No additional treatment needed.
Contributing factors: Water in the entryway.
Prevention: Mats in entryway to absorb water.
Next of kin/guardian notified/patient: No
Medical staff notified: Yes
Contact phone number: 123-123-1234
Other persons involved: None
Position: N/A
Medical report: Minor bruising, no treatment.
Designation: Accidental
Check the Signature on File box

1. Find the **Incident Form** in the **Form Repository**.

2. Complete all required fields. It is important to be specific and detailed in the documentation of an Incident Report.

3. Click the **Save** button.

An Incident Report is not part of the patient's medical record, so it is saved to a central location within the office rather than the patient record. In SimChart for the Medical Office, reference past incident reports by clicking the Saved Forms tab *(Figure 3-1)*. While it is not part of the patient record, it is still very important to document the incident accurately and objectively. The Incident Report is saved to be used as a tool to prevent the occurrence from happening again. It may be used to develop new policies and procedures to protect both patients and staff.

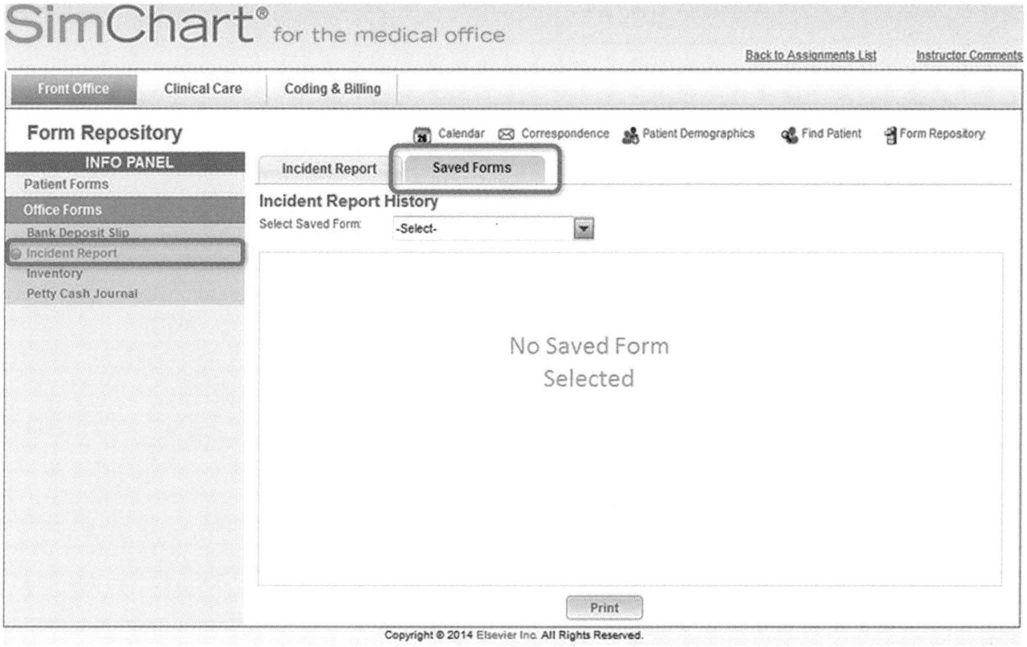

FIGURE 3-1 Incident Reports in the Saved Forms tab.

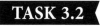

Referral Form

Another form that is often needed is a Referral Form. This form is used when one provider wants a patient to see another provider. It is often required by insurance carriers before they agree to pay for services provided by the new provider. Dr. Walden would like her patient Carl Bowden, DOB 04/05/1954, to see an endocrinologist for issues related to his type 2 diabetes. The endocrinologist is Dr. Casper at Anytown Endocrinology Clinic, 3661 Grant Avenue, Anytown, AL 12345. She would like to refer Carl for 10 visits.

Diagnosis: Type 2 diabetes, uncontrolled; ICD-9 250.02, ICD-10 E11.65
Significant clinical information/symptoms: Uncontrolled blood glucose
    levels, Hgb A1c 11.2%
Medications: Glimepiride 2 mg daily
Walden-Martin Family Medical Clinic, Phone 123-123-1234
Dr. Walden's NPI number: 987654321

✓ REFERRAL FORM

1. Find the **Referral** form in the **Form Repository** and perform a **Patient Search**.

2. Using the information provided above, complete all necessary fields.

3. Click the **Save to Patient Record** button.

Written Communication

Mora Siever missed her 3:30 appointment with Jean Burke, NP, yesterday afternoon. It is Walden-Martin Family Medical Clinic's policy to send a letter to patients who have missed an appointment. This serves two purposes. It documents the fact that the patient did not show up for a scheduled appointment and gives the patient the opportunity to reschedule the appointment. Jill would like you to generate a Missed Appointment letter for Mora.

✓ MISSED APPOINTMENT LETTER

1. Find the **Missed Appointment** letter in **Correspondence** and perform a **Patient Search**.

2. Complete all necessary fields.

3. Click the **Save to Patient Record** button.

TASK 3.4

Preparing a Superbill and Posting to the Ledger

Another important administrative function is completing the Superbill and Ledger to document the services provided for billing purposes. The provider may complete the Superbill or it may be the office staff's job to complete. The information from the Superbill is then posted to the account ledger where a running total of the charges for the services provided and payments made on the account are recorded.

Jill has been auditing patient accounts to make sure that all patient visits have been billed, and she has found a visit on 08/09/2013 for Dr. Martin's patient Amma Patel, DOB 01/14/1988, that has no Superbill or Ledger entries. She was seen for iron deficiency anemia and she did not make a payment that day. The Superbill and Ledger are found by clicking on the Coding and Billing module *(Figure 3-2)*.

> Previous balance: 0.00
> Services provided:
> Established patient, problem-focused office visit
> Insurance:
> Blue Cross Blue Shield
> 1234 Insurance Place
> Anytown, AL 12345
> Phone: 800-123-1111
> Amma is the insured, ID number is WMF456987123, Group number is MW55874.
> Condition is not related to employment, auto accident, or other accident.
> Diagnosis: Iron deficiency anemia; ICD-9 280.9, ICD-10 D50.9
> HIPAA form is on file, date 08/09/2013

✔ SUPERBILL

1. Click on the **Coding and Billing** tab, then **Superbill** from the information panel on the left side of the screen, and do a **Patient Search**.

FIGURE 3-2 Coding and Billing module.

2. Under the **Encounters Not Coded** grid, click on **Comprehensive Visit—Follow-up/ Established Visit 08/09/2013**. This will open up the Superbill.

3. Determine the charge for the office visit by clicking on the **Fee Schedule** link and locating the correct office visit type. Enter that amount in the **Today's Charges** field. Complete other information in step 1.

4. Click **Save** and **Next** to move to step 5.

5. Select the **ICD-9** or **ICD-10** radio button, depending on which is used, and enter the diagnosis in the correct field.

6. Enter the service provided. Click the **Save** button and the **Next** button twice to move to step 7.

7. Scroll to the bottom of page 4 and click the box to indicate that you are ready to submit the Superbill.

8. Select the **Yes** radio button in the **Signature on File** field, and enter today's date in the **Date** field.

9. Click on the **Submit Superbill** button.

✓ **LEDGER**

1. Select **Ledger** from the information panel on the left side.

2. Using the information from the **Superbill**, complete the required fields for the Ledger.

3. Click the **Save** button.

TASK 3.5

Preparing an Insurance Claim

The next step in the billing process is to prepare the insurance claim. This will allow the information to be submitted electronically to the insurance carrier for processing and payment. You will be using information from the Superbill and from the box below to complete the insurance claim process.

> Billing Provider Information:
> Julie Walden
> Walden-Martin Family Medical Clinic
> 1234 Anystreet
> Anytown, AL 12345-1234
> Phone: 123-123-1234

✓ CLAIM

1. Select **Claim** from the information panel on the left side of the screen and perform a **Patient Search**. You will see the encounter for DOS 08/09/2013 with the status of Not Started. Click on the paper and pencil icon to open the claim.

2. The claim consists of seven tabs. Review the autopopulated information for the Patient Info, Provider Info, Payer Info, Encounter Notes, and Claim Info tabs. Add any missing information and click the **Save** button for each tab.

3. On the **Charge Capture** tab, click the Place of Service link to determine the correct the POS (Place of Service) code. Click the **Save** button.

4. Click on the **Submission** tab and click the checkbox next to **I am ready to submit the Claim**.

5. Select the **Yes** radio button in the Signature on File field and enter **08/09/2013** in the Date field.

6. Click the **Submit Claim** button.

This has been another information-packed day! You have learned about risk management and have been introduced to the electronic billing process. Good work!

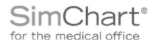
SimChart®
for the medical office

DAY FOUR

Task 4.1
Emailing Patients Regarding Test Results

Task 4.2
Handling Telephone
Messages and Scheduling
Appointments for Established Patients

Task 4.3
Scheduling New
Patient Appointments
and Generating Appropriate Forms

Task 4.4
Documents Received in the Mail

Task 4.5
Prior Authorization Request

TASK 4.1

Emailing Patients Regarding Test Results

There are many different ways of communicating information to patients. It can be done with a phone call, a traditional letter, or an email. The use of email to communicate with patients is on the rise in healthcare. In the past, email had not been considered confidential, and maintaining patient confidentiality is key in healthcare. However, more and more patients want to receive information quickly and in the format with which they are most comfortable, and for many that is email. In addition, as part of the Health Information Technology for Economic and Clinical Health (HITECH) Act and Meaningful Use, eligible professionals are required to use secure electronic messaging to communicate with patients regarding relevant health information. Jill explains to you that it is the policy of the Walden-Martin Family Medical Clinic to relay information to patients using the secure email system if the patient has given permission to do so. The patient must also supply the clinic with the proper email address to use. The patient will sign a form giving permission for emails to be sent to a specific email address. The patient can choose to use email for appointment reminders, normal laboratory test results, and answers to questions.

When Jon Wilson was in for his annual examination, Dr. Martin ordered a lipid profile based on Jon's family history of coronary artery disease. The results have come back from the outside laboratory and all are normal. Jon has given permission for his test results to be emailed to him and he would like a copy of the results sent as well. Jill asks that you send out the email with the results as an attachment.

✓ SENDING AN EMAIL WITH AN ATTACHMENT

The electronic health record has several templates already set up for the most common types of emails and letters that the clinic sends out. The normal test results template is one of these types.

1. Find the **Normal Test Results** template by clicking on the **Correspondence** icon *(Figure 4-1)*, locating the template, and performing a **Patient Search**.

2. Review the autopopulated fields and complete all other required fields.

3. Click on the **Attach File** button, then click on the **Browse** button and locate the laboratory results file (found on the Evolve website, Task 4.4; you must save this document to your computer or storage device before attaching it to this email). Click on the **Upload** button.

4. Click the **Send** button and a copy of the email will be saved to the patient record.

FIGURE 4-1 The Correspondence icon.

TASK 4.2

Handling Telephone Messages and Scheduling Appointments for Established Patients

Locate the **Telephone Messages** area on the companion Evolve website (Task 4.2). These are the nonurgent messages the clinic received last evening. As this is a task you have done before, Jill would like you to listen to the messages, complete a Phone Message for each in the electronic health record, schedule the appointment, and respond to the patient.

 PROFESSIONALISM

Email tips: Written communication is just as important as face-to-face communication. Maintaining a professional demeanor is harder to do when you do not have body language to help convey your message. It is important to proofread any written communication before it is sent out. If you are unsure that it conveys the message you really want, you should have someone else read it as well. If you are unsure about the spelling of any words, look them up in a dictionary. Do not completely rely on the software's spell-check as it will not indicate if you are using the word correctly (e.g., there, their, or they're).

✓ DOCUMENT PHONE MESSAGE, SCHEDULE APPOINTMENT, EMAIL PATIENT

1. Click on the **Correspondence** icon to locate **Phone Messages** on the left side of the screen *(Figure 4-2)* and perform a **Patient Search**.

2. Document the information accurately.

3. Schedule the appointment as close as possible to the time requested by the patient. Indicate the date and time of the appointment in the **Action Documentation** section of the **Phone Message**.

4. Click the **Save to Patient Record** button.

5. Using the **Blank Email** template, compose a professional email indicating the date and time the appointment has been scheduled, which doctor it is scheduled with, and how the patient should contact the office to change the appointment if the time is inconvenient.

6. Click the **Send** button.

7. You can view the email by clicking on **Find Patient**, doing a **Patient Search**, and then scrolling down to the **Correspondence** section of the Patient Dashboard.

Complete these steps for all messages remaining for this task.

SimChart® for the medical office

Front Office   Clinical Care   Coding & Billing

Correspondence   📅 Calendar   ✉ Correspondence   👥 Patient Demographics   🔍 Find Patient   📋 Form Repository

INFO PANEL
Emails
Letters
Phone Messages
⦿ Phone Messages

Phone Message

Please perform a patient search to find a specific patient.

WALDEN-MARTIN
FAMILY MEDICAL CLINIC
1234 ANYSTREET | ANYTOWN, ANYSTATE 12345
PHONE 123-123-1234 | FAX 123-123-5678

Date:		Time:
Caller:		Provider:
Regarding Patient:		Patient Date of Birth:

☐ PLEASE CALL   ☐ INFORMATION ONLY   ☐ RETURNED YOUR CALL   ☐ REQUEST

Message:

Pharmacy:

Provider Recommendation:

Action Documentation:

Completed By: Date/Time:

Patient Search   Print   Save to Patient Record   Cancel

Copyright © 2014 Elsevier Inc. All Rights Reserved.

FIGURE 4-2   Phone Messages in the Correspondence icon.

TASK 4.3

Scheduling New Patient Appointments and Generating Appropriate Forms

After taking care of the phone messages, Jill wants you to answer the telephone requests for appointments. Your first call is from a new patient requesting an appointment with Dr. Walden for an annual examination. Use the information below to schedule the appointment.

Patient name: Megan E. Adams
Date of birth: 09/27/1984
Address:
2310 Madison Avenue
Anytown, AL 12345
Phone: 123-435-5298
Emergency contact: Kevin Adams
Emergency contact phone: 123-435-6601
Employer: Anytown Hospital
Insurance:
Aetna
1234 Insurance Way
Anytown, AL 12345
Phone: 800-123-2222
Policy holder: Megan Adams
Social Security number: 444-92-5544
Policy/ID number: 0927198426
Group number: AH4218

Megan would like an appointment on any day at 11:00 AM. Access Dr. Walden's schedule and find an available day for this appointment. Remember that a new patient visit as well as an annual examination will take 45 minutes.

✔ SCHEDULE A NEW PATIENT APPOINTMENT

1. Open Dr. Walden's schedule.

2. Find the first 45-minute appointment available at 11:00 AM. Click on that time slot.

3. Enter the information necessary to add this patient and appointment. The appointment will appear on the calendar (refer to Task 1.4).

As with the previous new patient, Jon Wilson, whom you scheduled, you will need to send Megan the appropriate forms. Before doing so, you will need to complete the demographic information for Megan Adams. Using the information provided above, click on the **Patient Demographics** icon and complete the three tabs in this window (refer to Task 1.5).

✔ GENERATE APPROPRIATE FORMS

Using the **Correspondence** and **Form Repository** icons, complete the New Patient Welcome letter, Notice of Privacy Practice form, Patient Bill of Rights, and the Medical Records Release form. Save all of the documents to Megan's record.

To view the documents you have just created, click on the **Find Patient** icon and perform a **Patient Search** for Megan Adams. You will land on the Patient Dashboard of the electronic health record. By scrolling down the page, you will see the New Patient Welcome letter in the Correspondence section and the three forms you created in the Forms section. You can click on any of them to print them out if required by your instructor.

SCHEDULE A NEW PATIENT APPOINTMENT AND GENERATE APPROPRIATE FORMS

You take two more calls for new patients. Schedule the appointments using the information below.

Patient name: Thomas R. Carter
Date of birth: 02/24/1951
Address:
221 9th Street W.
Anytown, AL 12345
Phone: 123-467-9731
Emergency contact: Donna Carter
Emergency contact phone: 123-435-3621
Employer: Anytown Middle School
Insurance:
Aetna
1234 Insurance Way
Anytown, AL 12345
Phone: 800-123-2222
Policy holder: Thomas Carter
Social Security number: 777-32-1597
Policy/ID number: 0224195146
Group number: MS2264

Thomas would like an appointment on any day after 3:00 PM with Dr. Martin for a new patient visit to discuss his blood pressure. After the appointment has been scheduled, generate the appropriate forms for this new patient.

Patient name: Peggy Taylor
Date of birth: 01/12/1987
Address:
421 Main Street
Anytown, AL 12345
Phone: 123-552-1040
Social Security number: 989-22-8765
Emergency contact: Randy Taylor
Emergency contact phone: 123-552-6065
Employer: Anytown Accountants
Insurance:
Blue Cross Blue Shield
1234 Insurance Place
Anytown, AL 12345
Phone: 800-123-1111
Policy holder: Randy Taylor
Policy holder Social Security number: 898-44-6974
Policy/ID number: AAA587945
Group number: 45879FQ

Peggy would like an appointment anytime on a Thursday with Jean Burke, NP, for a new patient visit. After the appointment has been scheduled, generate the appropriate forms for this new patient.

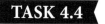

TASK 4.4

Documents Received in the Mail

With an electronic health record, many documents mailed to the clinic must be scanned and then uploaded to the medical record. Several documents have arrived in today's mail and have been scanned, and Jill would like you to upload them into the proper section of the patient's medical record.

✓ OPERATIVE REPORT

During her last visit with Dr. Martin, Norma Washington, DOB 08/01/1944, mentioned that she had a hip replacement several years ago when she lived elsewhere. Dr. Martin wanted to see the operative report for that procedure and asked Norma complete a Medical Records Release form. The operative report was received in the mail today and has been scanned. It now needs to be uploaded into the Health History section of Norma's record.

1. On the Evolve website, locate the documents for Task 4.4 and save them to your computer or storage device.

2. Click on the **Find Patient** icon and perform a **Patient Search**. The **Clinical Care** tab will open on the Patient Dashboard for Norma Washington.

3. To enter the health record, select the **Office Visit—Follow-up/Established Visit 08/15/2013** link within the **Encounters** section. The health record will open on the Allergies section displaying the **Record** drop-down menu *(Figure 4-3)*. Select **Health History** from the drop-down menu.

4. On the **Medical History** tab scroll down to **Past Surgeries** and click on the **Add New** button.

5. Enter the date of the surgery, found on the Operative Report, in the **Date** field. Enter "Left Hip Repair" in the **Type of Surgery** field.

SimChart® for the medical office

Back to Assignments List   Instructor Comments

| Front Office | Clinical Care | Coding & Billing |

Patient Charting

📅 Calendar   ✉ Correspondence   👥 Patient Demographics   🔍 Find Patient   📋 Form Repository

INFO PANEL

Washington, Nor...   ✖

Patient Dashboard

Washington, Norma B 08/01/1944   Expand

Office Visit

Follow-Up/Established Visit 08/15/2013 ▾   Add New   Record ▾

Phone Encounter

Allergies

	Allergies
	Chief Complaint
	Health History
	Immunizations
	Medications
	Order Entry
	Patient Education
	Preventative Services
	Problem List
	Progress Notes
	Vital Signs

Diagnostics / Lab Results

☐ No known allergies to drugs, foods, or environmental items

Showing 0 to 0 of 0 entries

Encounter Type	Type	Allergen	Reactions	Severity	Notes
No Data Saved					

Add Allergy   ☐ Reviewed   Upd

Save   Cancel

FIGURE 4-3   Record drop-down menu.

6. Click on the **Browse** button in the **Upload Surgical Record** section. Locate the previously saved Operative Report and click the **Save** button.

 ## IMMUNIZATION RECORD

Also in today's mail is an immunization record for Casey Hernandez, DOB 10/08/2000. This has been scanned and now needs to be uploaded to Casey's record.

1. Click on the **Find Patient** icon and perform a **Patient Search**. The Clinical Care tab will open on the Patient Dashboard for Casey Hernandez.

2. Enter the health record by clicking on the **Encounter**. Select **Immunizations** from the **Record** drop-down menu and upload the immunization record that you had previously saved from the Evolve website.

LABORATORY REPORT

In preparation for his upcoming annual examination with Dr. Martin, Jon Wilson, DOB 08/01/1986, has had his previously performed lipid profile results sent to the Walden-Martin Family Medical Clinic. These results have been scanned and now need to be uploaded to his record.

1. Click on the **Find Patient** icon and perform a **Patient Search**. The **Clinical Care** tab will open on the Patient Dashboard for Jon Wilson.

2. Select **Diagnostics/Lab Results** from the information panel on the left side of the screen and click the **Add** button.

3. Enter the date of the lipid profile from the report in the **Date** field.

4. Select the appropriate **Type** from the drop-down menu and indicate "lipid profile" in the **Notes** field.

5. Upload the report that you had previously saved from the Evolve website and click the **Save** button.

Prior Authorization Request

When Al Neviaser, DOB 06/21/1968, was in the office 3 days ago, he mentioned to Dr. Martin that he was having some lower back pain. Dr. Martin told him that if it did not get better, he would order an MRI to see what was going on. Al has called to say that the pain is actually getting worse. Jill tells you that because it is documented in the medical record that Dr. Martin would like to order an MRI, you should proceed with completing the Prior Authorization form.

Many insurance companies require prior authorization for certain services, including inpatient hospitalizations, new or experimental procedures, and certain diagnostic studies. Al's insurance carrier requires prior authorization for an MRI.

✓ **COMPLETE PRIOR AUTHORIZATION FORM**

1. Click on the **Form Repository** icon to locate the **Prior Authorization Request** and perform a **Patient Search**.

2. Use the information below to complete the form.

> Ordering physician: James A. Martin
> Provider contact name: Jill King
> Place of service/treatment and address:
> Anytown Hospital
> 2345 Anystreet
> Anytown, AL 12345
> Service requested: MRI of thoracic and lumbar spine
> Diagnosis/ICD code: Lower back pain ICD-9 724.2, ICD-10 M54.5
> Injury related?: No
> Workers' Compensation related: No

3. Click **Save to Patient Record**.

Once again, you have quickly and efficiently learned new skills. You have also been able to apply the skills that you have learned previously. You are well on your way to being a fantastic medical assistant!

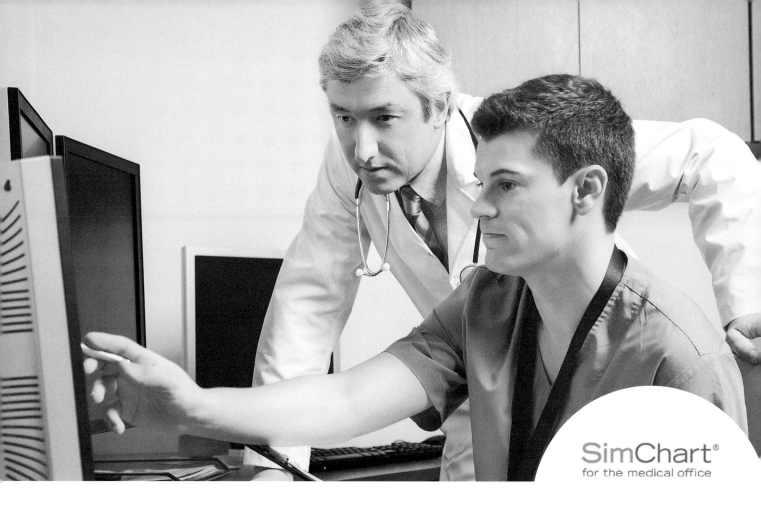

SimChart®
for the medical office

DAY FIVE

Task 5.1
Updating Patient Demographics

Task 5.2
Posting Charges to a Ledger

Task 5.3
Generating Patient Statements

Task 5.4
Completing a Day Sheet

Task 5.5
Preparing the Bank Deposit Slip

TASK 5.1

Updating Patient Demographics

Today Jill would like you to work in the billing department of the clinic. Correct billing is key to keeping the practice afloat financially. Attention to detail is especially important in this area.

You will start by updating demographics and then posting charges to patient ledgers. A patient ledger is where all financial activity for a patient is tracked. Any services or supplies that are given to a patient, any payments that are made, and any adjustments to the account are listed on the ledger, in which a running total of the account is kept.

People often move, change jobs, or change insurance carriers. All of these circumstances can impact billing. Patient statements need the correct patient address; insurance claims need the correct employer and insurance information. If the clinic does not have the correct information, billing can be delayed, which means there is a delay in reimbursement for the clinic. Jill has asked you to update the following patient demographic information.

Reuven Ahmad, DOB 09/12/1967, has been laid off by his employer. Reuven cannot afford to pay the insurance premium, even under COBRA, so he no longer has insurance.

1. Click on the **Patient Demographics** icon and perform a **Patient Search**.

2. Update the Guarantor and Insurance information.

3. Click the **Save Patient** button.

> **◎ PROFESSIONAL TIP**
>
> It is important to remain nonjudgmental when dealing with patients. When a patient has been laid off from his or her job and no longer has health insurance, the patient may feel badly about coming to the doctor. It is part of your job to make the patient feel as comfortable as possible in these circumstances. Having a list of community resources that may help is a good idea. The clinic may have a policy that will allow the patient to set up a payment plan to pay off the account over time. It is important to know the policies and procedures of the clinic when dealing with these sensitive situations.

Julia Berkley, DOB 07/05/1992, has moved to 125 1st Avenue, Anytown, AL 12345.

1. Click on the **Patient Demographics** icon and perform a **Patient Search**.

2. Update the appropriate fields.

3. Click the **Save Patient** button.

Quinton Brown, DOB 02/24/1978, now has insurance *(Figure 5-1)*.

1. Click on the **Patient Demographics** icon and perform a **Patient Search**.

2. Update the appropriate fields.

3. Click the **Save Patient** button.

MetLife   1234 Insurance Way

MEMBER NAME: Brown, Quinton

POLICY #: Q07976B

GROUP #: 35874B   **EFFECTIVE DATE:** 03/9/2013

CO-PAY: $25   DRUG CO-PAY
SPECIALIST CO-PAY: $35   GENERIC: $10
XRAY/LAB BENEFIT: $250   NAME BRAND: $50

CLAIMS/INQUIRIES: 1-800-123-4444

FIGURE 5-1   Quinton Brown's insurance card.

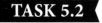

TASK 5.2

Posting Charges to a Ledger

Occasionally the clinic provides services that are not related to a medical condition. Charges for those services must be posted to the patient ledger. Previously you posted charges for medical services to a patient ledger. These charges will be posted in the same way.

 COPYING OF MEDICAL RECORDS

Monique Jones, DOB 06/23/1985, is planning an extensive trip to Europe and would like to have a copy of her medical records with her just in case she needs them. It is the policy at the Walden-Martin Family Medical Clinic to charge for records that are not being released to another provider or to the court. There will be a $5.00 charge for the copying and sending of the records.

1. Click on the **Coding and Billing** tab and then select **Ledger** from the information panel on the left side of the screen. Perform a **Patient Search**.

2. Using today's date and Medical Records for the service, post this charge to Monique's ledger.

3. Click the **Save** button.

 FORMS COMPLETION

Daniel Miller, DOB 03/21/2012, is going to be attending a new daycare. This new facility requires that a form be completed by the physician. There is a $10.00 fee for this service.

1. Locate the patient's **Ledger**. Notice that the Guarantor for this account is Chris Miller. As Daniel is a minor, he is not legally responsible for the bill. The guarantor is his parent.

2. Using today's date, post the charges for the form completion service to Daniel's ledger.

3. Click the **Save** button.

DAY FIVE TASK **5.2**

Generating Patient Statements

Another important part of the billing process is sending out patient statements. A statement can serve two purposes: it can let the patient know which services were provided and the fee for those services, and it can notify the patient of how much he or she owes the clinic.

Because the two services provided above are not covered by insurance, Jill has asked you to generate statements for those services to be sent to the patients.

✔ STATEMENT FOR MONIQUE JONES

1. Locate the **Patient Statement** in the **Form Repository** and perform a **Patient Search**.

2. Confirm the autopopulated fields.

3. Using today's date, complete the fields using Medical Records for the description. The full charge will be the patient's responsibility and should be paid in full by 1 month from today.

4. Click the **Save to Patient Record** button.

✔ STATEMENT FOR DANIEL MILLER

1. Complete the **Patient Statement** for Daniel.

2. Click the **Save to Patient Record** button.

Completing a Day Sheet

The Day Sheet is used to track all of the services that were provided and all of the payments received in the clinic on a given day. All charges, payments, and adjustments are listed along with the new balance on the patient account and the old balance (the balance prior to today's charges, payments, and/or adjustments) on the patient account. Jill has asked that you enter the following services and payments on the Day Sheet for today:

> Janine Butler: Services 99215 $75.00, 93000 $89.00; payment—check
>   (Patient Payment Check [PTPYMTCK]) $25.00; old balance $346.00
> Robert Caudill: Services 99203 $70.00, 69210 $46.00; payment—cash
> $10.00 (Patient Payment Cash [PTPYMTCS]); old balance $0.00
> Pedro Gomez: Services 99204 $89.00, 45330 $90.00; old balance $0.00
> Talibah Nasser: Services 99213 $43.00; payment—check (PTPYMTCK)
> $10.00; old balance $158.00
> Ella Rainwater: Services 99212 $32.00; old balance $35.00
> Kyle Reeves: Insurance payment (Insurance Payment [INSPYMT]) $120.00;
>   adjustment $35.00; old balance $155.00
> Ken Thomas: Insurance payment (INSPYMT) $550.00; adjustment $120.00;
>   old balance $820.00

✔ DAY SHEET ENTRIES

When posting to the Day Sheet *(Figure 5-2)*, one line is typically used for each patient (with last name listed first), so you should list all services provided in the services area of the Day Sheet separated by a comma, that is, 99213, 81000, and the total of all services in the Charges column. For insurance payments use the code INSPYMT in the Service column. You will have to calculate the new balance by starting with the old balance, adding in any charges and subtracting any payments and/or adjustments.

1. Click on the **Coding and Billing** tab to locate the **Day Sheet** on the left side.

2. Using the information provided above, enter all of the charges, payments, and adjustments for each patient on a separate line using the **Add Row** button as needed.

✔ DAILY PROOF OF POSTING; ACCOUNTS RECEIVABLE PROOF

To verify that all of the numbers have been entered correctly you will need to complete the Daily Posting Proof. The Accounts Receivable Proof provides the accounts receivable balance after the day's activities. This amount is carried forward to the next day's Day Sheet.

1. Using the column totals that have been autocalculated, complete the **Daily Posting Proof**. Your final total should match the total in Column D. If not, you will need to recheck the numbers entered into the Day Sheet. Make sure that your math was correct when adding the fees entered in the Charges column and when you calculated the New Balance.

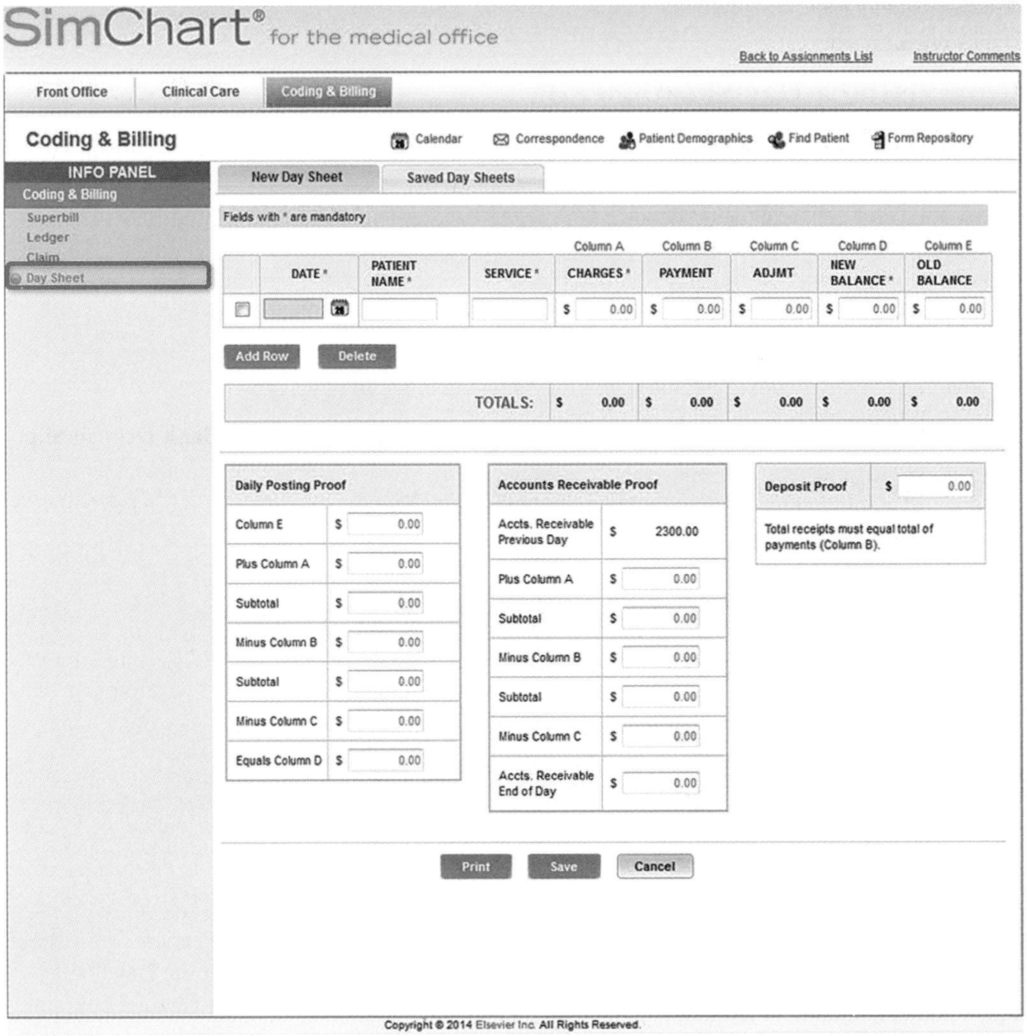

FIGURE 5-2 Day Sheet.

2. Complete the **Accounts Receivable Proof**.

3. Enter the amount from Column B in the **Deposit Proof**. This number should match the amount of the Deposit Slip.

4. Click the **Save** button.

Preparing the Bank Deposit Slip

At the end of the day, the last task in the business office is to prepare the bank deposit slip. All of the payments received for the day are listed on this slip. This slip along with the endorsed checks and any cash received are taken to the bank so that the funds can be deposited in the clinic's bank account.

 BANK DEPOSIT SLIP

1. Click on the **Form Repository** icon and then **Office Forms** to locate the **Bank Deposit Slip**.

2. Use the payments listed in Task 5.4 to complete the bank deposit slip, listing the patient's last name first.

3. Click the **Save** button.

You are halfway through your administrative practicum! You have accomplished so much in just 5 days. Give yourself a round of applause!

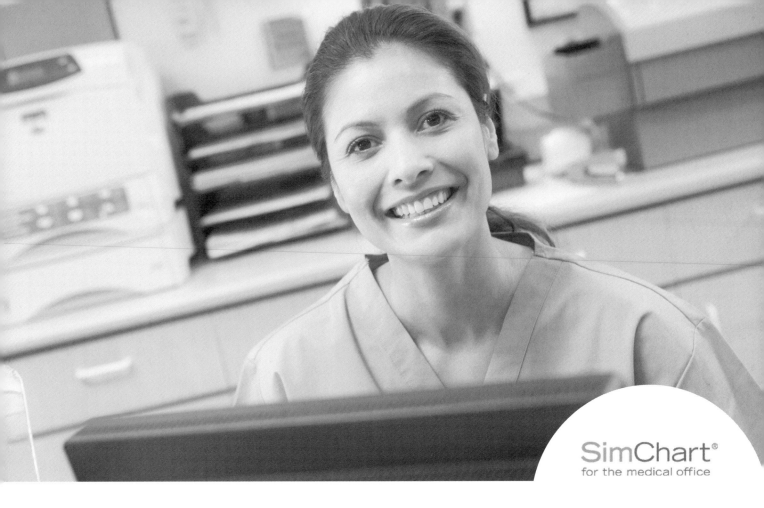

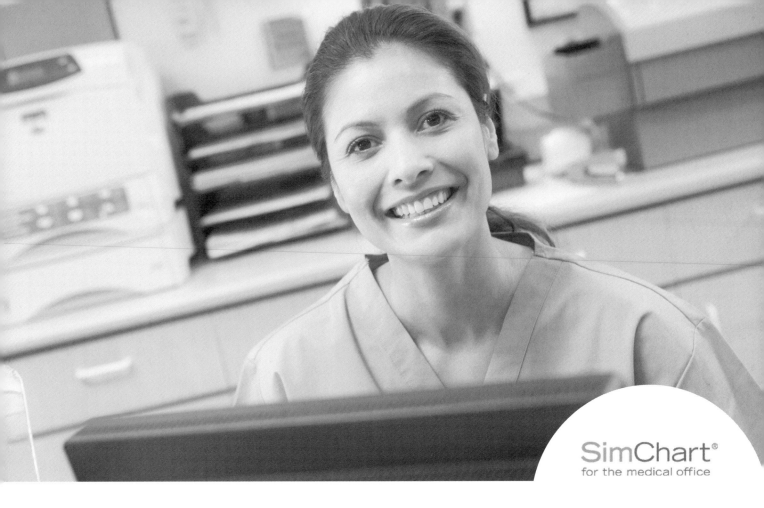

DAY SIX

Task 6.1
Collection Letter

Task 6.2
Denial Letter

Task 6.3
Insurance Claims Tracer

Task 6.4
Maintaining a Petty Cash Fund

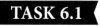

Collection Letter

You are back in the billing department today to learn more of what is involved in collecting funds for services rendered. One of those tasks is to send out collection letters for balances that have been outstanding for more than 60 days. It is the policy of the Walden-Martin Family Medical Clinic to give the patient 10 days to respond to a collection letter before further action is taken.

It has been discovered that Anna Richardson, DOB 02/14/1978, has an outstanding balance from DOS 08/09/2013. Her insurance made a payment but there is still a balance due that is her responsibility. Jill asks that you create the collection letter for this account.

✓ GENERATING A COLLECTION LETTER

To complete the collection letter, you will need to determine which services were provided and what the balance is on Anna's account. That information can be found on the Superbill and Ledger.

1. Click on the **Coding and Billing** tab and gather the necessary information from the **Superbill** and **Ledger**.

2. Click on the **Correspondence** icon, **Letters**, and **Collection**. Perform a **Patient Search**.

3. Verify autopopulated information and enter any additional information that is needed.

4. Click on the **Save to Patient Record** button.

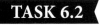

Denial Letter

The balance left on an account after the insurance has paid is sometimes the patient's responsibility due to the deductible not being met yet or coinsurance that is the patient's responsibility. Sometimes the balance is the patient's responsibility because the service has been denied by the insurance carrier. The patient may not realize that he or she is responsible for that balance. The Walden-Martin Family Medical Clinic has a policy to send letters to patients when services have been denied by their carriers so that they are aware that it is their responsibility. It is also part of that policy to allow a patient 30 days from the date of the letter to pay the outstanding balance.

In reviewing the accounts with outstanding balances, it is discovered that Norma Washington has an outstanding balance for a pap test performed on 08/15/2013. This service was denied by Medicare because Norma had a normal pap test the previous year and Medicare pays for a screening pap test only every 2 years. Jill asks that you create the denial letter for Norma Washington.

✓ GENERATING A DENIAL LETTER

To complete the denial letter, you will need to determine the balance on Norma's account.

1. Determine the balance on the account by viewing the **Ledger**.

2. Select the **Denial** letter template from the information panel on the left side of the screen and perform a **Patient Search**.

3. Verify the autopopulated information and enter any additional information that is needed.

4. Click on the **Save to Patient Record** button.

Insurance Claims Tracer

The majority of the income for any medical clinic comes from insurance reimbursement. It is important that all claims are paid in a timely fashion. To be sure that happens, the medical clinic must keep track of claims and follow up on those that are not paid in the expected time frame (10-14 days for an electronic claim, 30-45 days for a paper claim). If a claim is not paid in the expected time frame, an Insurance Claims Tracer can be used to follow up with the insurance carrier.

It has been discovered that a claim for Truong Tran, DOB 05/30/1991, for DOS 02/20/2014 has not been paid or denied. Jill asks that you prepare the Insurance Claims Tracer form.

✔ PREPARING THE INSURANCE CLAIMS TRACER FORM

To complete this form, you will need the account number from the Ledger and the charges, date, and diagnosis listed on the original claim.

1. Locate the **Insurance Claims Tracer** in the **Form Repository** and perform a **Patient Search**.

2. Confirm the autopopulated fields and complete all other fields.

3. Click the **Save to Patient Record** button.

TASK 6.4

Maintaining a Petty Cash Fund

Petty cash is a small amount of cash kept on hand to cover some of the everyday expenses that arise, such as parking, postage, or lunch for the doctor. While the name "petty cash" may lead you to believe that it is not very important, that would be an incorrect assumption. It is important to keep track of how those funds are used and also to make sure that there is actual cash in the petty cash fund for those minor expenses. Due to a turnover in staff at the Walden-Martin Family Medical Clinic, the petty cash fund has not been well managed lately. Jill asks that you take on that task to update it.

 PETTY CASH JOURNAL

When you open the lockbox that is used for the petty cash fund, you see that there are some receipts and $200 in cash. You also notice that no one has recorded anything in the petty cash journal *(Figure 6-1)* for last month. Your first step is to organize the receipts by date and then start the petty cash journal for last month.

FIGURE 6-1 Petty Cash Journal.

Dated the 18th, receipt for tissues and cotton balls purchased from the drug
    store, $15.89
Dated the 4th, receipt for postage due paid, $4.75
Dated the 26th, receipt for lunch for the doctor, $12.50
Dated the 12th, receipt for parking for a conference attended by the office
    manager in another city, $6.50

1. Locate the **Petty Cash Journal** form in the **Office Forms** section of the **Form Repository**.

2. Using the information provided above, post the items to the Petty Cash Journal, entering the dollar amounts in the correct column, using the **Add Row** button as needed. (Remember that all fields with an asterisk [*] are mandatory.)

3. Complete all other required fields, using today's date as the **Date Reconciled**.

4. Click the **Save** button.

You have had a couple of busy days in the billing department. You should now have a better understanding of how the billing process works to keep the money coming into the practice. You should also have a better understanding of how important it is to pay attention to the details. If you are off by one number, it can impact many areas of the reimbursement cycle.

You have been doing a great job. Keep up the good work!

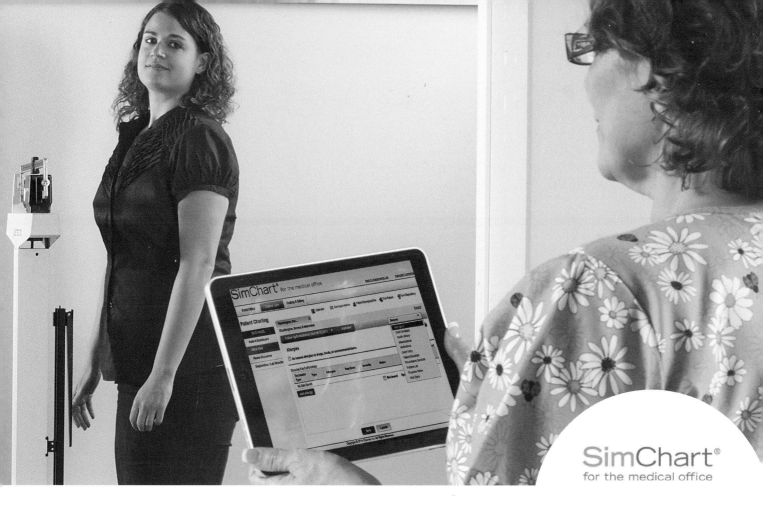

DAY SEVEN

Task 7.1
Establishing a Meeting

Task 7.2
Scheduling a Recurring Staff
Meeting with a Memorandum

Task 7.3
Scheduling Office Procedures
and Requesting Prior Authorization

Task 7.4
Using the Fee Schedule
and Responding to a Patient

Task 7.5
Patient Termination Letter

Today, Jill has given you some tasks to complete that are similar to tasks you have done before. For the scheduling tasks, Jill feels that you should be familiar enough with the process that she has given you just some basic information.

TASK 7.1

Establishing a Meeting

Your first task for today is to schedule a meeting for all three of the providers to discuss equipment purchases for the coming year. They would like the meeting to occur next week in the afternoon. You will then send a memorandum to all of the providers telling them the date and time of the meeting.

✓ SCHEDULING THE MEETING

1. Use the arrow keys on the **Calendar** to move to next week.

2. Locate a day and time, after lunch, when all three providers are available for 1 hour.

3. Schedule a **Block** appointment for all providers.

4. Click on the **Save** button.

✓ CREATING THE MEMORANDUM

1. Locate the **Email Memorandum** template in **Correspondence.**

2. The Memorandum is being sent to Dr. Walden, Dr. Martin, and Jean Burke, NP.

3. Complete all fields and compose a professional message containing all of the information about the meeting.

4. Click on the **Save** button.

PROFESSIONALISM

With so much of our personal communication happening in the electronic world, it is easy to let some of that style creep into our professional lives as well. It is important to keep electronic communication at work professional. Spelling and grammar are key components to professional communication. All words should be completely spelled out unless it is an accepted abbreviation. That means that "are" is spelled "are," not "R"; "you" is not "U"; and so on. If you are unsure about the spelling or grammar when sending an email, you can use the spell and grammar checker found in the email program or type it into a word processing program first. One caution, though: you should not rely solely on the spell checker, as it will tell you only if the word is spelled incorrectly, not if you have used it incorrectly; for example, to, too, and two are spelled correctly but have different meanings.

Scheduling a Recurring Staff Meeting with a Memorandum

The providers at the Walden-Martin Family Medical Clinic feel that it is important to bring the staff together for a meeting once a month to disseminate important information about changes or new policies within the clinic, discuss any issues that may have come up, and provide an opportunity for the staff to come together as a team. A memorandum needs to be sent to all of the staff telling them the day and time for the monthly meeting.

✔ SCHEDULING A RECURRING MEETING

Due to the providers' other commitments, such as hospital rounds, the meeting will need to be on Tuesdays at 2:00 PM. The only room large enough for all of the staff to meet in is the Meeting Room.

1. Locate next Tuesday on the **Calendar**.

2. Create the monthly recurring appointment in the **Meeting Room**.

3. Click on the **Save** button.

✔ CREATING THE MEMORANDUM

1. Locate the **Email Memorandum** template in **Correspondence**.

2. The memorandum is being sent to **All Staff**.

3. Complete all fields and compose a professional message containing all of the information about the meeting.

4. Click on the **Save** button.

Scheduling Office Procedures and Requesting Prior Authorization

There are several different office procedures that are done frequently at the Walden-Martin Family Medical Clinic. One procedure is a sigmoidoscopy, which takes 1 hour and is performed in Exam Room 1; another is a colposcopy, which takes 45 minutes and is performed in Exam Room 2. Dr. Martin has asked you to schedule one of his patients for a sigmoidoscopy, and Jean Burke, NP, has asked you to schedule one of her patients for a colposcopy with biopsy.

✔ SCHEDULING THE PROCEDURES

Charles Johnson, DOB 03/03/1958, needs to have a sigmoidoscopy scheduled. He is Dr. Martin's patient and would like to have this procedure done sometime next week when he can get an afternoon appointment.

use annual exam & procedure in chief complaint

1. Schedule Charles for the sigmoidoscopy procedure, making sure to designate the correct exam room and time for this procedure.

Noemi Rodriguez, DOB 11/04/1971, needs to have a colposcopy with biopsies scheduled. She is a patient of Jean Burke, NP, and would like to have this done as early in the day as possible on Thursday of next week.

1. Schedule Noemi for the colposcopy procedure, making sure to designate the correct exam room and time for this procedure.

✔ REQUESTING PRIOR AUTHORIZATION

Charles's insurance requires prior authorization for a sigmoidoscopy. Complete the appropriate form to request the prior authorization.

1. Locate the **Prior Authorization Request** form and perform a patient search.

2. Use the information below to complete the form.

> Ordering physician: James A. Martin
> Provider contact name: Jill King
> Place of service/treatment and address:
> Walden-Martin Family Medical Clinic
> 1234 Anystreet
> Anytown, AL 12345
> Service requested: Sigmoidoscopy
> Diagnosis/ICD code: Screening for malignant neoplasm of colon; ICD-9
>   V76.51, ICD-10 Z12.11
> Procedure/CPT code: 45330
> Injury related?: No
> Workers' Compensation related: No

3. Click the **Save to Patient Record** button.

Noemi's insurance also requires a prior authorization for a colposcopy. Complete the appropriate form to request the prior authorization.

1. Locate the **Prior Authorization Request** form and perform a patient search.

2. Use the information below to complete the form.

> Ordering physician: Jean Burke, NP
> Provider contact name: Jill King
> Place of service/treatment and address:
> Walden-Martin Family Medical Clinic
> 1234 Anystreet
> Anytown, AL 12345
> Service requested: Colposcopy with biopsies
> Diagnosis/ICD code: Cervical intraepithelial neoplasm II; ICD-9 622.12,
>   ICD-10 N87.1
> Injury related?: No
> Workers' Compensation related: No

3. Click the **Save to Patient Record** button.

Using the Fee Schedule and Responding to a Patient

Ken Thomas, DOB 10/25/1961, has emailed the clinic and is wondering what the cost of having a vasectomy is. He has requested a reply via email. Jill would like you to look up the fee for this procedure and then compose a professional email reply.

 FEE SCHEDULE

1. Click on the **Coding and Billing** tab to locate the link for the **Fee Schedule**.

2. Click on the link titled **Fee Schedule**.

3. Locate **Vasectomy** under **Office Procedures** and determine the fee.

 EMAIL

1. Find the **Blank Email** template by clicking on **Correspondence** and then perform a **Patient Search**.

2. Review the autopopulated fields and complete all other fields.

3. Compose a professional email stating the fee for the requested procedure.

◎ PROFESSIONALISM

Always keep in mind that you represent the clinic and providers for whom you work when you communicate with patients. The language used in an email to a patient should be as professional as the language you use to communicate with physicians and coworkers. Remember to use correct spelling and grammar. It is also important to remember to include a salutation and complimentary closing in a professional email.

---

4. Click the **Send** button, and a copy of the email will be saved to the patient record.

TASK 7.5

Patient Termination Letter

Celia Tapia, DOB 05/18/1970, a patient of Dr. Martin, has missed several appointments and is not responding to phone messages left for her. Jill explains that it is the policy of the Walden-Martin Family Medical Clinic to terminate the physician/patient contract when more than three appointments have been missed and there is no response from the patient. She asks you to create the Patient Termination letter to be sent to Celia.

 CREATING LETTER

1. Locate the **Patient Termination** letter template in **Correspondence** and do a **Patient Search**.

2. Review the autopopulated fields and verify that the date of termination is 30 days from today's date.

3. Click the **Save to Patient Record** button.

You have successfully completed your seventh day! You have learned much and are now applying it to new situations. You are using your critical thinking skills well.

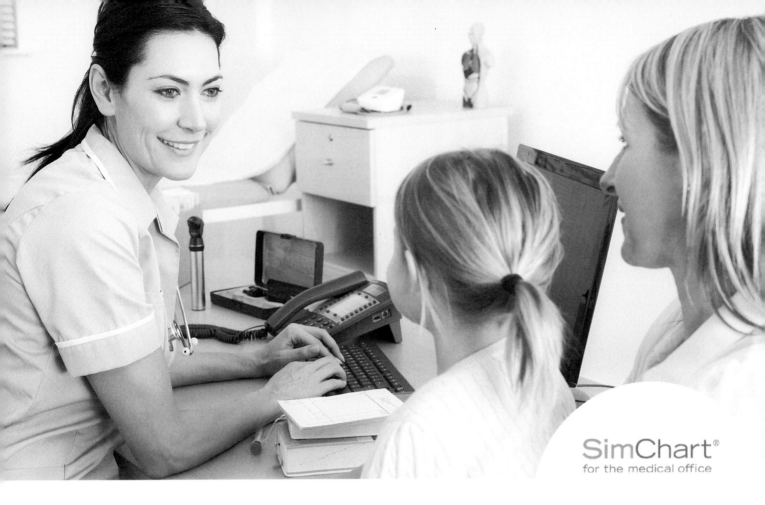

SimChart®
for the medical office

DAY EIGHT

Task 8.1
Inventory Management

Task 8.2
Certificate to Return to Work or School

Task 8.3
Memorandum Regarding Cell
Phone Use during Work Hours

Task 8.4
Walk-in Patients

Task 8.5
Telephone Messages

TASK 8.1

Inventory Management

To keep an office running smoothly and efficiently, there needs to be an adequate amount of supplies on hand to accomplish the tasks for the day. Inventory management is how an office knows when supplies are running low and when an order should be placed. Most offices make an inventory and order supplies on a set schedule. Some supplies may be ordered weekly and others may be ordered monthly or even quarterly. Jill would like you to take a look at the recent inventory that was made for the front office supplies and complete the inventory form. This information will be used to determine which supplies need to be ordered.

Table 8-1 shows the list of supplies with the quantity that is on hand. The reorder level is the point at which you need to order that particular supply. If there are seven of a particular item on hand and the reorder level is 10, that would indicate that you need to order more of that item. The quantity to reorder is how much of that supply should be ordered. You should order the full number of items listed in the quantity to reorder even though you still have some on hand. The number of items on hand should keep you supplied until the new order arrives.

✔ **INVENTORY FORM**

1. Locate the **Inventory** form in the **Form Repository** under **Office Forms**.

2. Using the information in Table 8-1, complete the form, using the **Add** button as needed to create additional rows.

3. Click the **Save** button.

✔ **PURCHASE ORDER**

1. Determine which supplies need to be ordered based on the quantity on hand and the reorder level listed in Table 8-1. If the quantity on hand is at or below the reorder level, it should be ordered.

TABLE 8-1 Supply List

	Quantity on Hand	Unit	Price/ Unit	Reorder Levels	Quantity to Reorder
Jumbo paper clips, smooth	4 boxes	box	$1.10	5 boxes	20 boxes
Staples, ¼ in.	5 boxes	box	$3.79	7 boxes	30 boxes
White-out correction fluid, 3/pack	4 bottles	pack	$3.99	2 packs	15 packs
Manila end tab file folders, letter size, 100/box	3 boxes	box	$17.99	2 boxes	25 boxes
Print or write multiuse ID labels, 3 in. H × 4 in. L, 80/pack	1 pack	pack	$6.99	1.5 pack	12 packs
AA alkaline batteries, 4/pack	6 each	pack	$4.99	1 pack	15 packs
3 in. × 5 in. line-ruled colored sticky notes, 5/pack	18 each	pack	$12.69	3 packs	2 packs
Paper clips, #1 size, nonskid	4.5 packs	pack	$6.14	5 packs	50 packs
Ballpoint pens, medium, black, dozen	11 each	dozen	$6.89	1 dozen	75 boxes

2. Locate the **Purchase Order** form in the **Form Repository** under **Office Forms** and print the blank form by clicking on the printer icon in the gray bar at the top of the form.

3. Using today's date and the information below, complete the top portion of the form.

Submitter: Walden-Martin Family Medical Clinic
PO number: 487762
Supplier: Anytown Office Supply
Phone: 123-123-9876
Website: www.anytownofficesupply.com

4. List the items you have determined should be ordered, including the quantity, unit, and price/unit.

5. Calculate the cost of ordering that item by multiplying the quantity by the price/unit and enter this amount in the **Cost** column.

6. When all of the items have been listed, add up the cost of each item to determine the total cost of the order and enter this amount in the **Total** field.

Certificate to Return to Work or School

Walter Biller, DOB 01/04/1970, a patient of Dr. Walden, needs to provide his employer with documentation that he is able to return to work after having broken his shoulder. It has been 8 weeks since the fracture, and Dr. Walden feels that he is completely healed and can return to work with no restrictions.

 COMPLETE THE CERTIFICATE TO RETURN TO WORK OR SCHOOL FORM

1. Locate the **Certificate to Return to Work or School** form in the **Form Repository** and do a **Patient Search**.

2. Review the autopopulated field and complete the other fields using the information provided above.

3. Click on the **Save to Patient Record** button.

TASK 8.3

Memorandum Regarding Cell Phone Use during Work Hours

There have been some issues with employees at the Walden-Martin Family Medical Clinic using their cell phones during the work day. Some of the patients have noticed it and commented on it to Dr. Walden. Dr. Walden brought it to Jill's attention, and she has asked you to prepare a memorandum using today's date from Jill King, Office Manager, to all employees about the policy regarding the use of cell phones during working hours. The memorandum should remind the staff that cell phones should not be answered during working hours except in the case of emergencies. Staff can carry their cell phones with them but they must be switched to silent mode. Cell phones should not be answered when working with patients. Texting and other cell phone activities should be limited to breaks and lunch times.

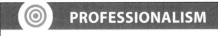 MEMORANDUM

1. Locate the **Memorandum** template from the **Email** section of **Correspondence** and create a professional email to all employees reminding them of the cell phone policy.

> **⊚ PROFESSIONALISM**
>
> In healthcare, it is important to keep things concise. This is true for professional correspondence as well as documentation in the health record. Your message should be clear and concise. Get to the point so you are not wasting anyone's time.

2. Click the **Send** button. A copy of the email will be saved and can be accessed by clicking on **Sent Memorandums**.

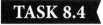

TASK 8.4

Walk-in Patients

While you are working at the front desk, one of your duties is to handle any patient issues that come up. One of the most common situations that comes up is the walk-in patient, a patient who does not have an appointment scheduled and wants to be seen today. Some patients should be seen on the same day if possible, such as those who have a fever, sore throat, or painful urination; others can wait until the next available time slot such as an annual examination or wellness visit.

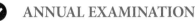 **ANNUAL EXAMINATION**

Jeffrey Raymond, DOB 09/25/1960, stops by the Walden-Martin Family Medical Clinic. He has heard fantastic things about Dr. Walden and would like to schedule an annual exam with her, today if possible. You ask Jeffrey to complete a patient registration form while you view the schedule.

1. Locate Dr. Walden's schedule and find the next available time slot for an annual exam (45 minutes).

2. Jeffrey agrees to the date and time that you have found, so you schedule his appointment.

3. Using the completed **Patient Information** form *(Figure 8-1)*, fully complete the patient demographics section.

FEVER AND SORE THROAT

Kay Peterson, DOB 08/06/1982, states that she has had a fever and sore throat for the past 2 days and really does not feel well. She is willing to see any provider if she can get an appointment today. You check the policy manual and you see that a fever and sore throat is listed under the conditions that should get a same-day appointment, even if it means double booking a provider. You have Kay complete a patient information form while you review the schedule.

1. Review the schedule and find the first available time slot (45 minutes) in today's schedule.

2. Kay agrees to the time you have available, so you schedule her appointment.

3. Using the completed **Patient Information** form, *(Figure 8-2)*, fully complete the patient demographics section.

WALDEN-MARTIN
FAMILY MEDICAL CLINIC
1234 ANYSTREET ANYTOWN, ANYSTATE 1234
PHONE 123-123-1234   FAX 123-123-5678

PATIENT INFORMATION

PATIENT INFORMATION (Please use full legal name.)

Last name: _Raymond_   Address 1: _916 Livingston Ln_

First name: _Jeffrey_   Address 2: _Anytown_

Middle initial: _S_   City: _AL_

Medical record number: _____   State: _12345_

Date of birth: _9/25/1960_   Zip: _____

Age: _53_   Email: _jraymond@wirefoxmail_

Sex: ☒ Male   ☐ Female   Home phone: _123-123-0449_

SSN: _987-23-5432_   Driver's license: _____

Emergency contact name: _Julie Raymond_   Emergency contact phone: _123-123-0449_

Mother's date of birth: _____   Father's date of birth: _____

Mother's work phone: _____   Father's work phone: _____

Mother's SSN: _____   Father's SSN: _____

Language: _English_   Race: _____

                                                 Ethnicity: _____

GUARANTOR INFORMATION (Please use full legal name.)

Relationship of guarantor to patient: ☒ Self   ☐ Spouse   ☐ Parent   ☐ Other

Guarantor/account #: _____

Account number: _____

Last name: _____   Address 1: _____

First name: _____   Address 2: _____

Middle initial: _____   City: _____

Date of birth: _____   State: _____

Age: _____   Zip: _____

Sex: _____   Email: _____

SSN: _____   Home phone: _____

Employer name: _Smith Electric_   Cell phone: _____

School name: _____   Work phone: _____

FIGURE 8-1   Jeffrey Raymond's Patient Information form.

OTHER EMPLOYMENT INFORMATION

Father's employer: _____   Mother's employer: _____

Employer's address 1: _____   Employer's address 1: _____

Employer's address 2: _____   Employer's address 2: _____

City: _____   City: _____

State: _____   State: _____

Zip: _____   Zip: _____

PROVIDER INFORMATION

Primary provider: _Dr. Walden_____   Provider's address 1: _1234 Anystreet_____

Referring provider: _____   Provider's address 2: _____

Date of last visit: _____   City: _____Anytown_____

Phone: _123-123-1234_____   State: _____AL_____

                                                 Zip: _____12345_____

INSURANCE INFORMATION (If the patient is not the Insured party, please include date of birth for claims.)

PRIMARY INSURANCE

Insurance: _Met Life_____   Claims address 1: _1234 Insurance Ave_____

Name of Policy Holder: _Jeffrey Raymond_____   Claims address 2: _____

SSN: _987-23-5432_____   City: _____Anytown_____

Policy/ID number: _L85027C_____   State: _____AL_____

Group Number: _40275M_____   Zip: _____12345_____

                                                 Claims phone: _800-123-4444_____

SECONDARY INSURANCE

Insurance: _____   Claims address 1: _____

Name of Policy Holder: _____   Claims address 2: _____

SSN: _____   City: _____

Policy/ID number: _____   State: _____

Group Number: _____   Zip: _____

                                                 Claims phone: _____

"I hereby authorize direct payment of all insurance benefits otherwise payable to me for services rendered. I understand that I am financially responsible for all charges not covered by insurance for services rendered on my behalf to my dependents. I authorize the above providers to release any information required to secure payment of benefits. I authorize the use of this signature on all insurance submissions."

Signature: _____JS Raymond_____   Date: _____

FIGURE 8-1, cont'd

WALDEN-MARTIN
FAMILY MEDICAL CLINIC
1234 ANYSTREET ANYTOWN, ANYSTATE 1234
PHONE 123-123-1234   FAX 123-123-5678

PATIENT INFORMATION

PATIENT INFORMATION (Please use full legal name.)

Last name: _Peterson_   Address 1: _457 College Ave_

First name: _Kay_   Address 2: _____

Middle initial: _M_   City: _Anytown_

Medical record number: _____   State: _AL_

Date of birth: _08/06/1982_   Zip: _12345-1234_

Age: _____   Email: _kay@wirefox.mail_

Sex: ☐ Male   ☒ Female   Home phone: _123-123-6798_

SSN: _123-45-9876_   Driver's license: _AL535311_

Emergency contact name: _Cathy Peterson_   Emergency contact phone: _123-123-5421_

Mother's date of birth: _____   Father's date of birth: _____

Mother's work phone: _____   Father's work phone: _____

Mother's SSN: _____   Father's SSN: _____

Language: _Spanish and English_   Race: _Mexican_

                                                     Ethnicity: _Hispanic_

GUARANTOR INFORMATION (Please use full legal name.)

Relationship of guarantor to patient: ☒ Self   ☐ Spouse   ☐ Parent   ☐ Other

Guarantor/account #: _____

Account number: _____

Last name: _____   Address 1: _____

First name: _____   Address 2: _____

Middle initial: _____   City: _____

Date of birth: _____   State: _____

Age: _____   Zip: _____

Sex: _____   Email: _____

SSN: _____   Home phone: _____

Employer name: _Anytown Library_   Cell phone: _123-123-6667_

School name: _____   Work phone: _123-123-4501_

FIGURE 8-2   Kay Peterson's Patient Information form.

OTHER EMPLOYMENT INFORMATION

Father's employer: _____   Mother's employer: _____

Employer's address 1: _____   Employer's address 1: _____

Employer's address 2: _____   Employer's address 2: _____

City: _____   City: _____

State: _____   State: _____

Zip: _____   Zip: _____

PROVIDER INFORMATION

Primary provider: _____   Provider's address 1: _____

Referring provider: _____   Provider's address 2: _____

Date of last visit: _____   City: _____

Phone: _____   State: _____

                                              Zip: _____

INSURANCE INFORMATION (If the patient is not the Insured party, please include date of birth for claims.)

PRIMARY INSURANCE

Insurance: _Aetna_____   Claims address 1: _1234 Insurance Way_____

Name of Policy Holder: _Kay Peterson_____   Claims address 2: _____

SSN: _____   City: _Anytown_____

Policy/ID number: _B24892N_____   State: _AL_____

Group Number: _42856M_____   Zip: _12345_____

                                              Claims phone: _800-123-2222_____

SECONDARY INSURANCE

Insurance: _____   Claims address 1: _____

Name of Policy Holder: _____   Claims address 2: _____

SSN: _____   City: _____

Policy/ID number: _____   State: _____

Group Number: _____   Zip: _____

                                              Claims phone: _____

"I hereby authorize direct payment of all insurance benefits otherwise payable to me for services rendered. I understand that I am financially responsible for all charges not covered by insurance for services rendered on my behalf to my dependents. I authorize the above providers to release any information required to secure payment of benefits. I authorize the use of this signature on all insurance submissions."

Signature: _Kay Peterson_____   Date: _____

FIGURE 8-2, cont'd

TASK 8.5

Telephone Messages

Locate the "Telephone Messages" area on the companion Evolve website (Task 8.5). These are the nonurgent messages that came into the clinic over the lunch hour. Jill would like you to listen to the messages, complete a Phone Message for each in the electronic health record, schedule appointments (if necessary), and respond to the patient.

◎ PROFESSIONALISM

Phone messages can be left for a number of different reasons: medical questions for the physicians; requests for procedures, lab results, or prescription refills; billing questions; or general questions. Some of these can be handled by the medical assistant, such as general billing questions, directions to the clinic, or scheduling appointments, but some need to be handled by the physician, such as questions regarding care and treatment, requests for new prescriptions, or complications from a procedure. If you are unsure whether you can take care of the situation, ask your supervisor.

✔ DOCUMENT PHONE MESSAGE, SCHEDULE APPOINTMENT, EMAIL PATIENT

1. Locate **Phone Messages** in **Correspondence** and perform a **Patient Search**.

2. Document the information accurately.

3. If necessary, schedule the appointment as close as possible to the time requested by the patient. Indicate the date and time of the appointment in the **Action Documentation** section of the **Phone Message**.

4. Click the **Save to Patient Record** button.

5. If an appointment has been scheduled, use the template to compose a professional email indicating the date and time the appointment has been scheduled for, which doctor it is scheduled with, and how the patient should contact the office to change the appointment if the time is inconvenient.

◎ PROFESSIONALISM

Email correspondence and interoffice messaging are often used to communicate within the medical clinic. It is important to maintain patient confidentiality in all correspondence. It may be the policy to use only a patient identification number in correspondence within the clinic. You should be knowledgeable of the clinic's policies regarding email communication.

---

6. Click the **Send** button. You can view the email by clicking on the **Find Patient** icon, performing a **Patient Search**, and then scrolling down to the **Correspondence** section.

Complete these steps for all messages remaining for this task.
    Only 2 days left in your practicum! Keep up the good work!

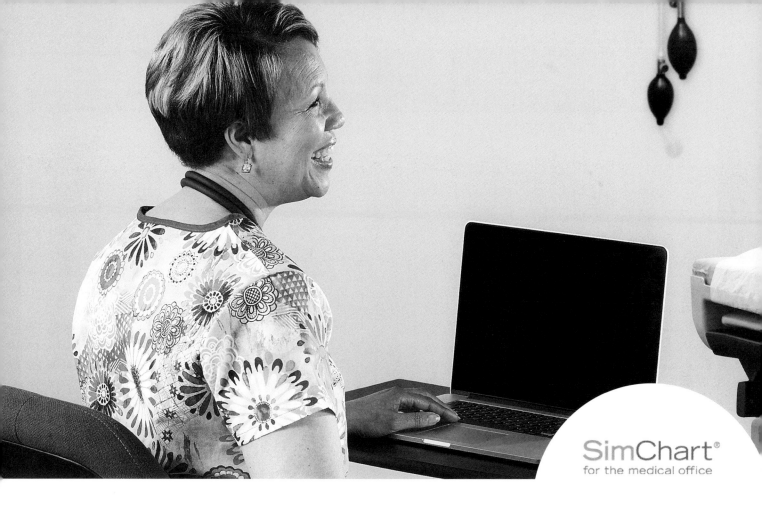

DAY NINE

Task 9.1
Next available apt

Scheduling New Patient Appointments

Task 9.2
Screen shot dashboard only

Generating Appropriate
Forms for a New Patient

Task 9.3

Scheduling Appointments for Established
Patients

Task 9.4

Correcting Demographic Information

Task 9.5

Creating a Referral Request

You are starting your ninth day in your practicum and Jill feels that you can work fairly independently. You will be working on tasks that you have done previously.

TASK 9.1

Scheduling New Patient Appointments

Your first task today is to schedule a new patient for an annual examination with Dr. Walden. Judy Merrill calls and requests an appointment on a Monday morning with Dr. Walden. In this situation you should use New Patient for the visit type and Annual Exam as the reason for the visit. Use the information below to schedule her appointment (refer to Box 1-1 for length of appointment).

Patient name: Judy M. Merrill
Date of birth: 05/21/1960
Insurance:
Aetna
1234 Insurance Way
Anytown, AL 12345
Phone: 800-123-2222
Policy holder: Judy Merrill
Social Security number: 322-88-3922
Policy/ID number: P78549S
Group number: 45789R

✔ SCHEDULE A NEW PATIENT APPOINTMENT

1. Open Dr. Walden's schedule and find the correct day and time.

2. Schedule the appointment for the appropriate amount of time (refer to Box 1-1).

You have asked Judy if she has time to give you the rest of her demographic information, and she has said yes, she does.

◎ PROFESSIONALISM

When working in a busy medical clinic it is easy to get distracted. It is important to stay focused on the patient at all times even when on the phone. By having your work station completely supplied with things like pens, scratch paper, clock, or watch, you can complete a phone call without having to search for a pen to write down a phone message. Patients can tell, even on the phone, if they do not have your complete attention. Eating, drinking, or chewing gum can all be sensed by the person on the other end of the phone call. You will have a much more satisfied patient if you make that phone call your priority.

✓ COMPLETE DEMOGRAPHIC INFORMATION

Use the information below to complete the Patient Demographics section of the electronic health record for Judy Merrill.

Patient name: Judy M. Merrill
Date of birth: 05/21/1960
Address:
922 Old Farm Road
Anytown, AL 12345
Phone: 123-455-9246
Emergency contact: Pete Merrill
Emergency contact phone: 123-455-5823
Language: English
Race: White
Ethnicity: Not Hispanic or Latino
Employer: Anytown Law Firm
Insurance:
Aetna
1234 Insurance Way
Anytown, AL 12345
Phone: 800-123-2222
Policy holder: Judy Merrill
Social Security number: 322-88-3922
Policy/ID number: P78549S
Group number: 45789R

1. Click on the **Patient Demographics** icon and complete a **Patient Search**.

2. Enter all of the required information on the three tabs.

TASK 9.2

Generating Appropriate Forms for a New Patient

As Judy is a new patient of the Walden-Martin Family Medical Clinic, you will need to send her all the forms required.

 GENERATE APPROPRIATE FORMS

1. Using the **Correspondence** and **Form Repository** icons, complete the **New Patient Welcome** letter, **Notice of Privacy Practices**, **Patient Bill of Rights**, and the **Medical Records Release**.

2. **Save** all of the documents to Judy's record.

To view the documents you have just created, click on the Find Patient icon and perform a Patient Search for Judy Merrill. You will land on the Patient Dashboard of the electronic health record. By scrolling down the page, you will see the New Patient Welcome letter in the correspondence section and the three forms you created in the Forms section. You can click on any of them to print them out if required by your instructor.

TASK 9.3

Scheduling Appointments for Established Patients

Mrs. Burgel is calling to schedule a well-child visit for her daughter Isabella Burgel, DOB 07/23/2010. Isabella is an established patient of Dr. Martin and her mother is requesting an appointment for next Thursday in the early afternoon.

 ISABELLA BURGEL

1. Find the appropriate date and time for this appointment on Dr. Martin's schedule and perform a **Patient Search**.

2. Add the appointment for the appropriate length of time to Dr. Martin's schedule (refer to Box 1-1).

3. Click the **Save** button.

Maude Crawford, DOB 12/22/1946, has also called to schedule an appointment for a recheck of her blood pressure. She is Dr. Martin's patient but has heard such good things about Jean Burke that she would like to see her for this visit.

⊚ PROFESSIONALISM

Sometimes the smallest of gestures can make a patient's visit an exceptional visit. By saying please and thank you and having a smile on your face, patients will feel like the clinic is a pleasant place to be and that you really care about them. It takes very little time on your part to be courteous and friendly, but it can make a big difference in how patients view their visits to the clinic.

 MAUDE CRAWFORD

1. Find the appropriate date and time for this appointment on Jean Burke's schedule and perform a **Patient Search**.

2. Add the appointment for the appropriate length of time to Jean Burke's schedule (refer to Box 1-1).

3. Click the **Save** button.

TASK 9.4

Correcting Demographic Information

Patient demographic information can come to the medical office in several different ways. The patient may provide it directly or it may arrive from a different source, such as a returned letter from the U.S. Postal Service. Having the correct patient demographic information is key to billing correctly. Having accurate and complete demographic information allows for timely filing of claims and collection of insurance payments for the medical office. Jill has asked you to update the following patient's demographic information.

✅ UPDATING PATIENT DEMOGRAPHICS

The statement that was mailed to Jana Green, DOB 05/01/1936, has been returned to the Walden-Martin Family Medical Clinic by the post office with a change of address label on it. It appears that Jana has moved into an apartment. Her new address is 851 University Drive, Apt 322, Anytown, AL 12345-1322.

1. Click on the **Patient Demographics** icon and perform a **Patient Search**.

2. Update the patient's address.

3. Click the **Save Patient** button.

When you make an appointment reminder phone call to Janine Butler, DOB 04/25/1968, you get a recorded message that states her phone number has changed to 123-492-2155.

1. Click on the **Patient Demographics** icon and perform a **Patient Search**.

2. Update the appropriate fields.

3. Click the **Save Patient** button.

Truong Tran, DOB 05/30/1991, has called the office to say that he has a new job at Anytown Fitness and also that his insurance information has changed *(Figure 9-1)*.

1. Click on the **Patient Demographics** icon and perform a **Patient Search**.

2. Update the appropriate fields.

3. Click the **Save Patient** button.

MetLife	1234 Insurance Avenue
MEMBER NAME: Tran, Truong	
POLICY #: T18937T	
GROUP #: 64711K	**EFFECTIVE DATE:** 03/9/2013
CO-PAY: $25	DRUG CO-PAY
SPECIALIST CO-PAY: $35	GENERIC: $10
XRAY/LAB BENEFIT: $250	NAME BRAND: $50
CLAIMS/INQUIRIES: 1-800-123-4444	

FIGURE 9-1 Truong Tran's insurance card.

TASK 9.5

Creating a Referral Request

Dr. Walden would like her patient Erma Willis, DOB 12/09/1947, to be seen by a neurosurgeon for issues related to worsening migraine symptoms. The neurosurgeon requested by Dr. Walden is Dr. Randall at Anytown Neurology Associates, 9075 Hillview Road, Anytown, AL 12345. She would like to refer Erma for five visits.

> Diagnosis: Persistent migraine with aura, without cerebral infarction, intractable, without status migranosus; ICD-9 346.51, ICD-10 G43.519
> Significant clinical information/symptoms: headache pain with aura for 3 weeks
> Medications: Imitrex 50 mg
> Walden-Martin Family Medical Clinic, phone 123-123-1234
> Dr. Walden's NPI number: 987654321

✅ REFERRAL FORM

1. Find the **Referral** form in the **Form Repository** and perform a **Patient Search**.

2. Using the information provided above, complete all necessary fields.

3. Click the **Save to Patient Record** button.

Jill is very impressed with your work today! You have completed all of your tasks in a timely fashion. Keep up the good work! One more day to go!

DAY TEN

Task 10.1
Creating a Prior Authorization Request

Task 10.2
Creating the Superbill

Task 10.3
Posting to the Ledger

Task 10.4
Creating a Claim

Task 10.5
Completing the Day Sheet

This is the last day of your administrative practicum! Yesterday, you mostly worked on the scheduling tasks found in a medical office. Today, Jill would like you to work on the billing tasks.

PROFESSIONALISM

As you complete your practicum, it is important to keep in mind those things that employers are looking for above and beyond knowledge of how a medical clinic works. During your practicum, your supervisors and mentors are also looking for enthusiasm and a positive attitude. These attributes go a long way toward making a team function well. They are also evaluating your work ethic. Did you take the initiative to find something to do when you had completed a given task? Did you ask what else you could do? Did you arrive on time every day or even a little early? Any practicum experience is a chance for you to show all aspects of you. It is very much an extended job interview, even if that organization is not hiring. You should be confident to ask anyone with whom you worked to be a reference, which will help you obtain a position in your chosen career.

TASK 10.1

Creating a Prior Authorization Request

Two established patients of the Walden-Martin Family Medical Clinic need prior authorization for procedures. Jill has asked you to complete these requests.

✔ REQUESTING PRIOR AUTHORIZATION

Diego Lupez, DOB 08/01/1982, would like to have a vasectomy performed. Before scheduling the procedure, Dr. Martin has asked that you complete the Prior Authorization Request so that Diego can find out whether his insurance carrier will pay for the procedure.

1. Locate the **Prior Authorization Request** form and perform a **Patient Search**.

2. Use the information below to complete the form.

> Ordering physician: James A. Martin
> Provider contact name: Jill King
> Place of service/treatment and address:
> Walden-Martin Family Medical Clinic
> 1234 Anystreet
> Anytown, AL 12345
> Service requested: Vasectomy
> Diagnosis/ICD code: ICD-9 V26.52, ICD-10 Z98.52
> Procedure/ CPT code: 55250
> Injury related?: No
> Workers' Compensation related: No

3. Click the **Save to Patient Record** button.

REQUESTING PRIOR AUTHORIZATION

Celia Tapia, DOB 05/18/1970, needs to have an ingrown toenail removed. Celia is concerned that this will not be covered by her insurance Dr. Martin has asked that you complete the Prior Authorization Request so that Celia knows before the procedure is scheduled whether her insurance carrier will pay for this procedure.

1. Locate the **Prior Authorization Request** form and perform a **Patient Search**.

2. Use the information below to complete the form.

> Ordering physician: James A. Martin
> Provider contact name: Jill King
> Place of service/treatment and address:
> Walden-Martin Family Medical Clinic
> 1234 Anystreet
> Anytown, AL 12345
> Service requested: Nail removal with matrix
> Diagnosis/ICD code: Ingrowing nail; ICD-9 703.0, ICD-10 L60.0
> Procedure/ CPT code: 11750
> Injury related?: No
> Workers' Compensation related: No

3. Click the **Save to Patient Record** button.

Creating the Superbill

The Superbill for the wellness visit of Isabella Burgel, DOB 07/23/2010, needs to be completed. Use the information below and the fee schedule to complete the Superbill.

Previous balance: $0.00
Services provided: Established patient, well visit, 1-4 y
Isabella's mother, Amanda Burgel, is the insured, ID number is
    WMF456987123, Group number is 65321B.
Condition is not related to employment, auto accident, or other accident.
Diagnosis: Routine child check; ICD-9 V20.0, ICD-10 DZ00.129
HIPAA form is on file. Date: Today's date

✓ SUPERBILL

1. Click on the **Coding and Billing** tab, select **Superbill** from the information panel, and perform a **Patient Search**.

2. Under the **Encounters Not Coded** grid, click on the **Wellness Exam**. This will open up the Superbill.

3. Determine the charge for the office visit by clicking on the **Fee Schedule** link and locating the office visit. Enter that amount in the **Today's Charges** field. Complete any other necessary information on screen 1.

4. Click the **Save** button and then the **Next** button to move to screen 2.

5. Enter the diagnosis in the correct field indicating whether ICD-9 or ICD-10 codes are used.

6. Enter the service provided. Click the **Save** button, then the **Next** button twice to move to screen 4.

7. Scroll to the bottom of screen 4 and click the box to indicate that you are ready to submit the Superbill, select the **Yes** radio button for **Signature on File**, and today's date in the **Date** field.

8. Click on the **Submit Superbill** button.

Posting to the Ledger

The next step in the billing process is to post the charges to the ledger. Using the information from the Superbill, post the charges to the ledger for Isabella Burgel.

✓ **LEDGER**

1. Click on **Ledger** on the left side.

2. Using the information from the **Superbill**, complete the required fields for the ledger.

3. Click the **Save** button.

TASK 10.4

Creating a Claim

After posting the charges to the ledger, the next step is to create a claim.

✅ **SUPERBILL**

1. Click on **Claim** on the left side, perform a **Patient Search** if necessary, and you will see the encounter. Click on the paper and pencil icon to open the claim.

2. There are seven tabs for the claim. Review the autopopulated information for the five Patient Info, Provider Info, Payer Info, Encounter Notes, and Claim Info tabs. Add any missing information. Click the **Save** button for each tab.

3. On the **Charge Capture** tab, the **POS** (Place of Service) code can be found by clicking on the **Place of Service** link. Enter all necessary information. Click the **Save** button.

4. Click on the **Submission** tab and click the checkbox next to **I am ready to submit the Claim**.

5. Select the **Yes** radio button for **Signature on File** and enter today's date in the **Date** field.

6. Click the **Submit Claim** button.

TASK 10.5

Completing the Day Sheet

Your last task is to complete the Day Sheet. Jill has asked that you enter the following services and payments on the Day Sheet for today:

- Isabella Burgel: Services 99392 $75.00; old balance $346.00
- Tai Yan: Services 99205 $119.00, 93000 $89.00; payment $10.00; old balance $0.00
- Aaron Jackson: Services 99392 $75.00, 90471 $10.00, 90633 $33.00; old balance $0.00
- Norma Washington: Services 99212 $32.00; payment $10.00; old balance $158.00
- Anna Richardson: Services 99395 $80.00; old balance $35.00
- Johnny Parker: Insurance payment (INSPYMT) $137.30; adjustment $12.23; old balance $137.30
- Walter Biller: Insurance payment (INSPYMT) $157.90; adjustment $35.00: old balance $820.00

 DAY SHEET ENTRIES

Using one line for each patient, post the CPT codes in the Service column and use the code INSPYMT for insurance payments in the Service column. You will have to calculate the new balance by starting with the old balance, adding any charges, and subtracting any payments and/or adjustments.

1. Click on the **Coding and Billing** tab to locate the **Day Sheet** on the left side.

2. Using the information provided above, enter all of the charges, payments, and adjustments for each patient on a separate line, using the **Add Row** button as needed.

✔ **DAILY PROOF OF POSTING; ACCOUNTS RECEIVABLE PROOF**

To verify that all of the numbers have been entered correctly, you will need to complete the Daily Posting Proof. The Accounts Receivable Proof provides the accounts receivable balance after the day's activities. This amount is carried forward to the next day's Day Sheet.

1. Using the column totals that have been autocalculated, complete the **Daily Posting Proof**. Your final total should match the total in Column D. If not, you will need to recheck the numbers entered into the Day Sheet. Make sure that your math was correct when adding the fees entered in the Charges column and calculating the New Balance.

2. Complete the **Accounts Receivable Proof**.

You have completed the last task for the practicum. You have impressed Jill and all of the providers at the Walden-Martin Family Medical Clinic with your attention to detail and ability to stay on task. The skills you have learned while at the clinic will serve you well in your chosen career.

Congratulations!